EXERCISES IN
DIAGNOSING ECG TRACINGS

EXERCISES IN DIAGNOSING ECG TRACINGS

MARY BOUDREAU CONOVER, R.N., B.S.

Instructor and Education Consultant,
California Hospital Medical Center,
Los Angeles, California; Instructor of Intermediate and
Advanced Arrhythmia Workshops,
West Hills Hospital, Canoga Park, California;
Education Consultant, Holy Cross Hospital Cardiac
Arrhythmia Center, Mission Hills, California

THIRD EDITION

with 699 illustrations

The C. V. Mosby Company

ST. LOUIS • TORONTO • PRINCETON   1984

MOSBY

A TRADITION OF PUBLISHING EXCELLENCE

Editor: Michael R. Riley
Assistant editor: Bess Arends
Manuscript editor: Stephen C. Hetager
Cover design: Suzanne Oberholtzer
Book design: Jeanne Bush
Production: Susan Trail

THIRD EDITION

The C.V. Mosby Company
11830 Westline Industrial Drive, St. Louis, Missouri 63146

Library of Congress Cataloging in Publication Data

Conover, Mary Boudreau
   Exercises in diagnosing ECG tracings.

   Rev. ed. of: Cardiac arrhythmias. 2nd ed. 1978.
   1.   Electrocardiography—Problems, exercises, etc.
2.   Cardiovascular disease nursing—Problems, exercises,
etc.   I.   Conover, Mary Boudreau, 1931-   Cardiac
arrhythmias.   II.   Title.   [DNLM: 1.   Arrhythmia—Programmed
texts.   2.   Electrocardiography—Programmed texts.   WG 18
C753ea]
RC683.5.E5C645   1984   616.1'207'547076   84-3289
ISBN 0-8016-1238-1

C/VH/VH   9   8   7   6   5   4   3   2   1   03/B/324

To the critical care nurses
of America

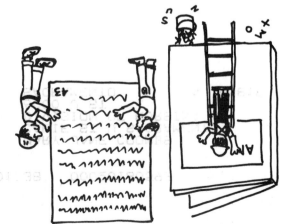

HELP US BUILD BETTER BOOKS

Meeting your needs is our business. You can help us meet these needs by sharing your opinions with us. This **MOSBY/TIMES MIRROR** text has been sent to you with our compliments. We hope you'll share in our enthusiasm over this excellent text. Please share your opinions with us. . .We need you to help us build better books!

Title: CONOVER EXERCISE ECG 3

P44 050184 01238 0002016059 31

MARY JANE COOMBS
CALIF ST U SACRAMENT
DIVISION OF NURSING
6000 J ST
SACRAMENTO   CA 95819

1. Is this book suitable for your course(s)?
   Yes _____
   No _____

2. If yes, do you plan to adopt this book?
   Yes _____
   No _____   How many? _____

3. Please identify some of the features that lead you to select this text for your course(s).
   a.) _____
   b.) _____
   c.) _____

4. If you have chosen not to adopt this text, please explain any deficiencies you may have encountered:
   Content _____   Comprehension Level/Too High _____
   Presentation _____   Comprehension Level/Too Low _____
   Comments: _____

5. What book(s) are you now using in your course?
   _____
   _____

   Why did you choose this book?
   _____
   _____

6. If you have not yet adopted a textbook for your course, what is your decision date? _____

Your comments are welcome. We rely on you to help us build better MOSBY/TIMES MIRROR BOOKS!

Please write: Marketing Services
MOSBY/TIMES MIRROR
11830 Westline Industrial Drive
St. Louis, MO 63146

Or Call: (800) 325-4177 ext. 588
In Missouri call collect:
(314) 872-8370 ext. 588
Would you be willing to discuss this questionnaire with us? If so, please indicate your phone number. _____

Fold, moisten and mail.

PRINTED BY THE STANDARD REGISTER COMPANY U.S.A. STANSET ®

115397

PREFACE

This book offers a simplified and rapid approach to ECG interpretation. Each chapter begins with programmed instruction, which is followed by enough actual ECG tracings to give you the practice you need and to make you feel comfortable with a particular diagnosis.

As you begin a chapter, study the details of each illustration and read the legend. Cover the answers on the right side of the page and read each statement, filling in the missing word or words. Then check your answers. Each statement is calculated to help you understand the mechanism of an arrhythmia and to give you the clues you need for a quick diagnosis.

By the time you have studied all of the illustrations at the beginning of the chapter, you will have enough knowledge to proceed with the practice tracings. Again, cover the right side of the page. After you have made your own measurements and diagnosis, read the diagnosis provided. If your diagnosis is incorrect, do not be discouraged. With each practice tracing there are instructions on the fastest and simplest way to a correct diagnosis of that particular arrhythmia. Continue on and you will be challenged by the same arrhythmia again and by different arrhythmias. Each tracing is chosen to provide you with the building blocks to a quick and correct conclusion.

Each chapter is carefully planned so that the diagnosis of ECG tracings may be learned in a systematic manner, with each chapter building on the previous one.

This book can be used alone or with two companion books for a complete home study program. The companion books are a more detailed textbook, *Understanding Electrocardiography: Arrhythmias and the 12-Lead ECG*, fourth edition, and a study guide, *Electrocardiography: A Home Study Course*.

Mary Boudreau Conover

CONTENTS

1

ARRHYTHMIAS ORIGINATING IN THE SINUS NODE

- ☐ **Sinus tachycardia**
- ☐ **Sinus bradycardia**
- ☐ **Sinus arrest**
- ☐ **SA block**
- ☐ **SA reentry**
- ☐ **Sick sinus syndrome**

Normal sinus rhythm

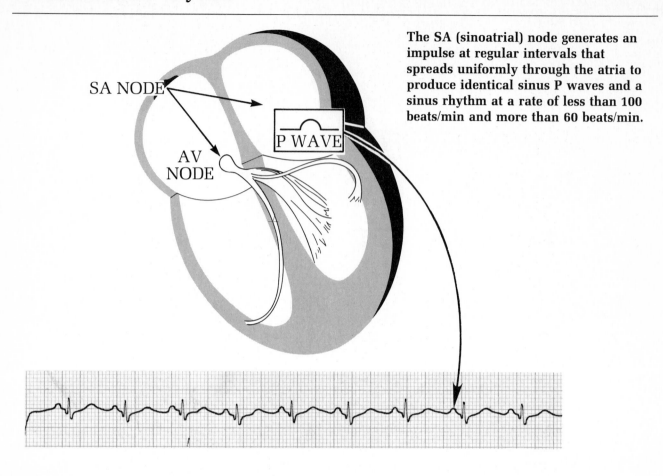

The SA (sinoatrial) node generates an impulse at regular intervals that spreads uniformly through the atria to produce identical sinus P waves and a sinus rhythm at a rate of less than 100 beats/min and more than 60 beats/min.

SA NODE

AV NODE

P WAVE

The sinus P waves are usually _____.   **regular**

The _____ _____ paces the heart.   **SA node**

The sinus P waves in one lead are _____.   **identical**

NOTE: The sinus rhythm may be influenced by respiration, especially in the young; the sinus rate speeds up with inspiration and slows down with expiration. This is called a sinus arrhythmia.

Parasympathetic nerve supply

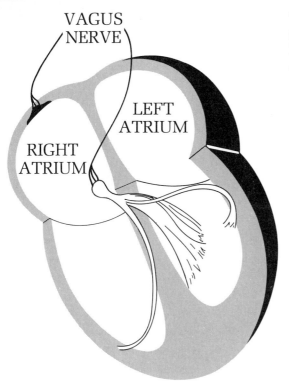

VAGUS NERVE

LEFT ATRIUM

RIGHT ATRIUM

The VAGUS nerve supplies both the SA and the AV (atrioventricular) nodes. When the heart rate increases or decreases, so does AV conduction time.

The SA and AV nodes respond _____ to the physiological needs of the body.

together

When the SA node speeds up, conduction time through the AV node is _____.

shorter

When the SA node slows down, conduction time through the AV node is _____.

longer

AV conduction

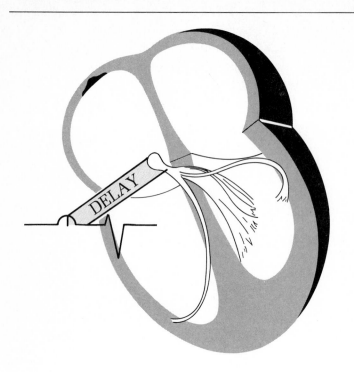

There is a delay in conduction through the AV node to allow for the "atrial kick" (atrial contribution to left-ventricular end-diastolic pressure).

The current from the SA node reaches the _____ _____ about midway through the P wave.

AV node

After a conduction delay in the AV node the impulse reaches the _____.

ventricles

Electrical activation of the ventricles produces the _____ complex.

QRS

ECG intervals

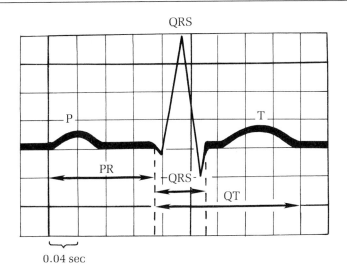

The PR, QRS, and QT intervals are important measurements.

On the horizontal plane each small square of the graph represents _____ sec.

0.04

The PR interval is measured from the beginning of the P wave to the beginning of the _____.

QRS

The QRS interval represents ventricular depolarization time; if it is narrow (less than 0.11 sec), conduction has begun above the branching of the bundle of His. Therefore the rhythm is _____.

supraventricular

The QT interval represents the ventricular refractory period and is measured from the beginning of the _____ to the end of the T wave.

QRS

Normal values for ECG intervals

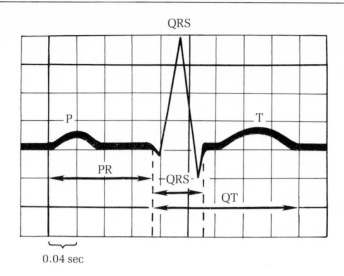

The PR interval should not be less than 0.12 nor more than 0.20 sec; the QRS duration should not exceed 0.11 sec; the QT interval changes with heart rate, but generally speaking should be less than half the preceding RR interval at rates between 65 and 90 beats/min (see Appendix).

A PR interval of 0.18 sec is (normal; abnormal).	**normal**
A PR interval of 0.22 sec is (normal; abnormal).	**abnormal**
A PR interval of 0.09 sec is (normal; abnormal).	**abnormal**
A QRS of 0.18 sec is (normal; abnormal).	**abnormal**
A QRS of 0.08 sec is (normal; abnormal).	**normal**

Regular rhythm

WHEN THE RHYTHM IS REGULAR

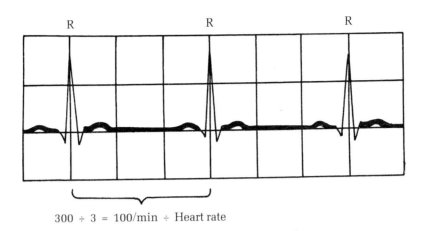

300 ÷ 3 = 100/min ÷ Heart rate

heart rate can be determined at a glance.

One way to determine heart rate when the rhythm is regular is to count the large squares between _____ _____.

R waves

Then, divide this number into _____.

300

300 ÷ Number of large squares between R waves = Heart rate

300 ÷ 3 = _____

100 beats/min

300 ÷ 2 = _____

150 beats/min

300 ÷ 4.5 = _____

66 beats/min

300 ÷ 5 = _____

60 beats/min

Irregular rhythm

WHEN THE RHYTHM IS IRREGULAR

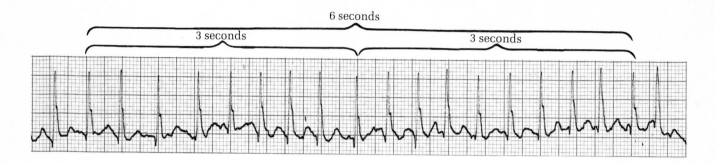

heart rate can be determined by counting the R waves in a 6-sec strip and multiplying by 10.

The ECG paper is divided along the top into _____-sec intervals. **3**

In this rhythm strip there are _____ R waves in a 6-sec strip. **18**

The approximate heart rate in the rhythm strip above is _____ beats/min. **180**

Tracing 1-1

V₁

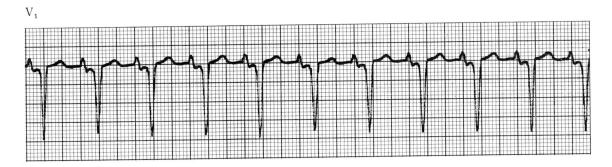

Rate: _____ beats/min   **100**

PR interval: _____ sec   **0.14**

QRS duration: _____ sec   **0.09**

QT interval: _____ sec   **0.30**

Conclusion: _____   **Sinus tachycardia**

In the setting of the coronary care unit, when the patient is at rest, a rate of 100 should elicit a physical assessment. Sinus tachycardia is a normal response to the body's demand for increased cardiac output. It is often the first sign of congestive heart failure, cardiogenic shock, pulmonary embolism, or infarct extension, and occurs with exercise, emotion, pain, fever, hyperthyroidism, or any condition that increases sympathetic stimulation.

Tracing 1-2

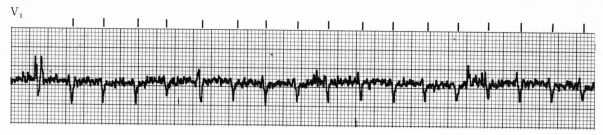

V₁

Artifact does not disturb the underlying rhythm.

Rate: _____ beats/min   **170**

PR interval: _____ sec   **Unknown**

QRS duration: _____ sec   **0.08**

QT interval: _____ sec   **Unknown**

Conclusion: _____   **Artifact**

Apart from the fact that this is a supraventricular tachycardia, artifact makes it impossible to interpret any further. Artifact is anything on the ECG tracing that has not been produced by the heart, whether it is a pacemaker blip, hiccoughs, alternating current (AC) interference, or the tremor from another muscle other than the heart (somatic tremor). The artifact above is caused by a loose electrode. The disturbance should obviously be corrected so that a proper interpretation can be made of the ECG.

Tracing 1-3

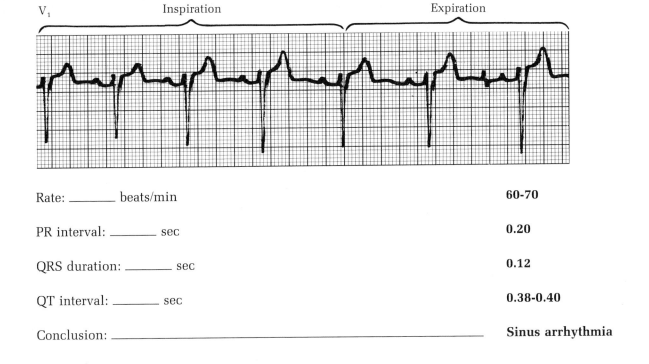

Rate: _____ beats/min   **60-70**

PR interval: _____ sec   **0.20**

QRS duration: _____ sec   **0.12**

QT interval: _____ sec   **0.38-0.40**

Conclusion: _____   **Sinus arrhythmia**

There are four things to notice in this tracing:
1. Sinus arrhythmia
2. Respiratory variations
3. An artifact
4. The QRS is too long.

The sinus arrhythmia is related to respiration. Notice that the RR intervals are gradually lengthening as the expiration phase of respiration begins. This has no clinical significance unless the bradycardia phase is profound and the patient is experiencing hemodynamic symptoms. In some cardiac arrhythmias, the bradycardia phase can be so slow as to allow a junctional escape beat.

The height of the S wave is also changing as a result of respiration (respiratory variations).

Toward the end of the tracing there is an artifact. It is a blip that does not belong to, nor does it influence, the cardiac rhythm; that is, it does not reset the sinus node or cause a P wave to be nonconducted.

Tracing 1-4

Alternating current

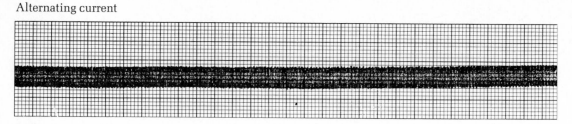

II

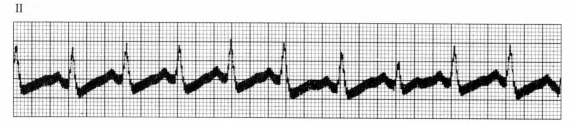

Rate: _____ beats/min

100

PR interval: _____ sec

Approximately 0.16

QRS duration: _____ sec

Approximately 0.12

QT interval: _____ sec

Unknown

Conclusion: _____

Artifact

These two tracings are presented to illustrate the effect of AC on the graph without (top) and with a concurrent ECG. The source of the interference should be identified and corrected. A 60-cycle AC artifact will always display an absolutely regular wave form that makes exactly 60 deflections/ sec. This regular type of artifact is easily differentiated from the erratic artifact of patient movement (somatic tremor).

AC interference on the tracing can result from several causes and may or may not represent a hazard to the patient. The situation should be corrected at once. If it is not due to a dry electrode pad or a defective patient cable, then defective electrical equipment in use on the patient should be suspected.

Tracing 1-5

II

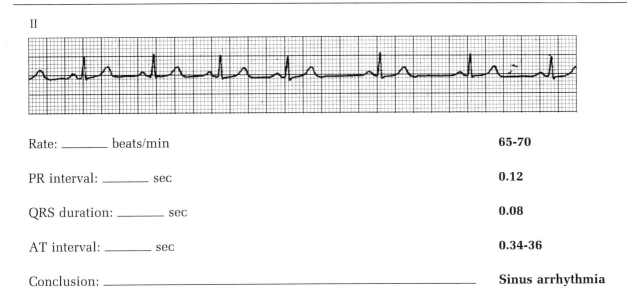

Rate: _____ beats/min   **65-70**

PR interval: _____ sec   **0.12**

QRS duration: _____ sec   **0.08**

AT interval: _____ sec   **0.34-36**

Conclusion: _____   **Sinus arrhythmia**

The pacemaker is the sinus node, and conduction is normal. The rhythm is irregular in that it gradually slows down and then speeds up again. This is normal and is related to respiration. If the difference between the shortest RR interval and the longest RR interval is greater than 0.12 sec, the rhythm qualifies as a sinus arrhythmia. In this tracing that difference is 0.26 sec.

Note the difference between the first QT interval and the last one. The QT accompanying the longer cycle is 0.02 sec. longer than that of the shorter cycle. This is because the refractory period changes with heart rate, becoming longer with bradycardia and shorter with tachycardia. The QT interval coincides with the cardiac action potential from phase 0 to the end of phase 3.

Tracing 1-6

V₁

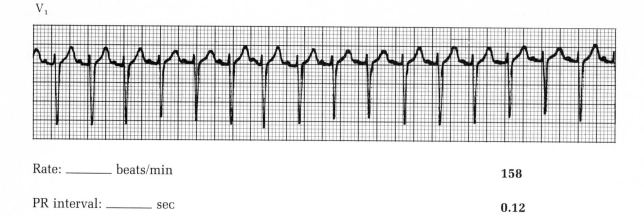

Rate: _____ beats/min   **158**

PR interval: _____ sec   **0.12**

QRS duration: _____ sec   **0.08**

QT interval: _____ sec   **0.26**

Conclusion: _____   **Sinus tachycardia**

A supraventricular tachycardia is certainly less serious than a ventricular tachycardia. However, it has been shown in animals and in humans that atrial pacing rates of greater than 120 to 140 beats/min will cause a significant decrease in coronary arterial blood flow. If such a rate is allowed to continue in a patient with acute myocardial infarction, a profound deficiency in coronary perfusion may result. This in turn would aggravate ischemia, allowing the ventricles to become more vulnerable to ventricular fibrillation and cardiac arrest.

As stated in the discussion of Tracing 1-1, sinus tachycardia may be the first sign of congestive heart failure. You should certainly question the need for the sinus node to beat that fast when the patient is at rest. Sinus tachycardia itself is not treated; it is necessary to determine and then treat the cause.

Tracing 1-7

II

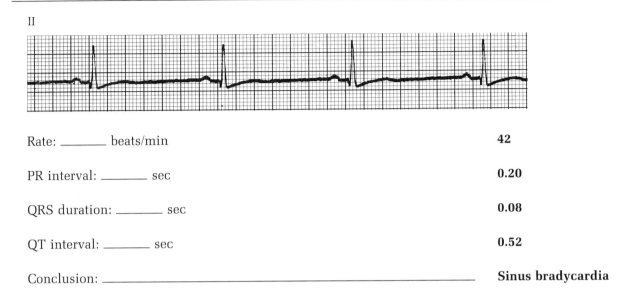

Rate: _____ beats/min   **42**

PR interval: _____ sec   **0.20**

QRS duration: _____ sec   **0.08**

QT interval: _____ sec   **0.52**

Conclusion: _____   **Sinus bradycardia**

   This is a sinus bradycardia (heart rate less than 60 beats/min). AV conduction is normal (the PR interval), and so is intraventricular conduction. The QT interval appears to be too long, but it is difficult to make this measurement; perhaps another lead would offer a more defined end to the T wave. A prolonged QT indicates lengthening of the refractory period, which may be secondary to quinidine or quinidine-like drugs, myocardial ischemia, or hypocalcemia. Hypokalemia causes a U wave, which may appear to lengthen the QT interval.

   Patients with sinus bradycardia usually have a benign clinical course. No treatment is required for this arrhythmia unless it is complicated by hypotension, or evidence of pump failure. In such a case steps should be taken to increase the heart rate.

Tracing 1-8

V₁

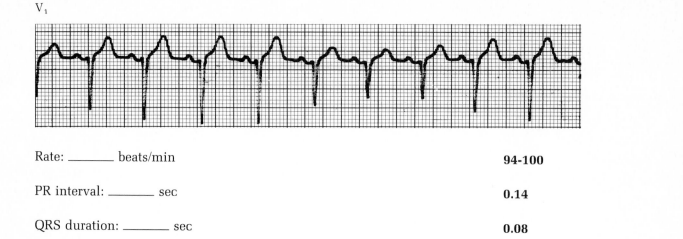

Rate: _____ beats/min   94-100

PR interval: _____ sec   0.14

QRS duration: _____ sec   0.08

QT interval: _____ sec   0.34

Conclusion: _____   **Normal sinus rhythm**

The narrow QRS complexes immediately identify this complex as supraventricular and the regular, uniform P waves as sinus. There is a slight increase in rate toward the end of the tracing, but not enough to call the rhythm a sinus arrhythmia. The respiratory variations are marked. With deep inspiration the heart position becomes more vertical, and with deep expiration more horizontal. The rotation of the heart is also affected; it rotates more clockwise during inspiration and counterclockwise during expiration.

Note that the QT interval is easy to measure in this tracing. When making this measurement, do not forget to take in the first part of the QRS, a little r wave.

Tracing 1-9

II

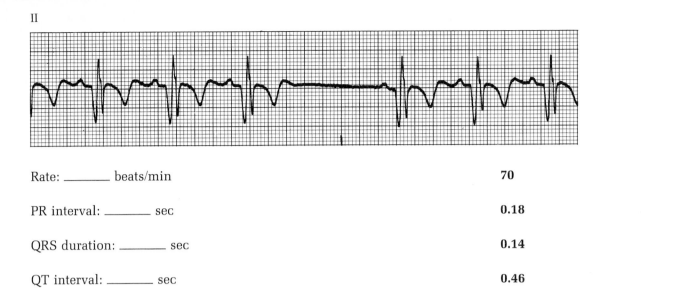

Rate: _____ beats/min   **70**

PR interval: _____ sec   **0.18**

QRS duration: _____ sec   **0.14**

QT interval: _____ sec   **0.46**

Conclusion: _____   **SA block or sinus
                                              arrest**

Sinus arrest and exit block of the sinus node (SA block) cannot always be distinguished from each other in the ECG. The mechanism of sinus arrest is depression of impulse formation, whereas the mechanism of SA block is depression of impulse conduction. In the above tracing one or the other has occurred spontaneously during a sinus rhythm. There is also a differential diagnosis between SA block or sinus arrest and a nonconducted premature atrial complex (PAC). This diagnosis is made by carefully examining the T wave preceding the pause and comparing it with the other T waves. If it shows any distortion at all, a hidden PAC is most probably the cause (see Chapter 2). The diagnosis is also made in light of the clinical setting.

Tracing 1-10

II

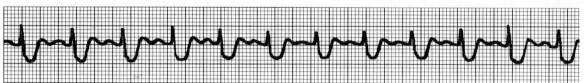

Rate: _____ beats/min   **110**

PR interval: _____ sec   **0.20**

QRS duration: _____ sec   **0.08**

QT interval: _____ sec   **0.32**

Conclusion: _____   **Sinus tachycardia**

Notice the scooped, pulled-down look of the ST segment, a typical digitalis effect. Myocardial ischemia will also cause the ST segment to be depressed. However, in the case of ischemia the QT interval would be prolonged, whereas digitalis causes a shortening. This is a helpful point to remember in the differential diagnosis of ST segment depression.

The clinical implications of sinus tachycardia have already been discussed in connection with Tracings 1-1 and 1-6.

Tracing 1-11

V$_1$

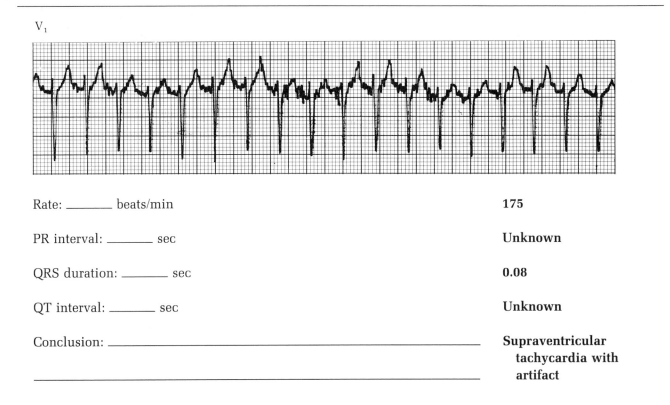

Rate: _____ beats/min

PR interval: _____ sec

QRS duration: _____ sec

QT interval: _____ sec

Conclusion: _____

_____

175

Unknown

0.08

Unknown

Supraventricular tachycardia with artifact

This is a supraventricular tachycardia. Somatic tremor makes any further evaluation of the tracing impossible. Notice the difference between the irregular, erratic artifact of this muscle tremor and the absolute regularity of AC interference (see tracing on p. 12)

Tracing 1-12

V_1

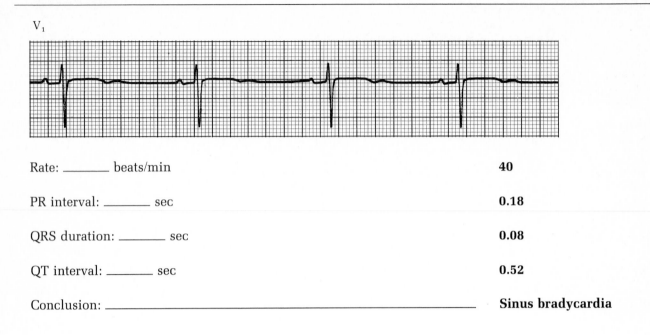

Rate: _____ beats/min   **40**

PR interval: _____ sec   **0.18**

QRS duration: _____ sec   **0.08**

QT interval: _____ sec   **0.52**

Conclusion: _____   **Sinus bradycardia**

A positive U wave is easily seen in this tracing. It is the extra little hump after the T wave. These are seen in normal people and become prominent in hypokalemia. The ECG is a very sensitive indicator of the ratio of intracellular to extracellular potassium and shows signs of hypokalemia even when the serum potassium level is still within normal limits.

Tracing 1-13

II

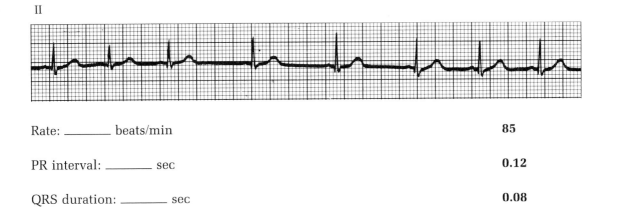

Rate: _____ beats/min   **85**

PR interval: _____ sec   **0.12**

QRS duration: _____ sec   **0.08**

QT interval: _____ sec   **0.32**

Conclusion: _____   **Sinus arrhythmia**

Since there is a difference of 0.32 sec between the shortest and the longest cycle, this qualifies as a sinus arrhythmia. The tracing was taken from a healthy 4-year-old boy, and this particular arrhythmia is almost always present in well children. The person who is accustomed to looking at the adult ECG will be very surprised to see such a degree of sinus arrhythmia so consistently in the child.

Tracing 1-14

V₁

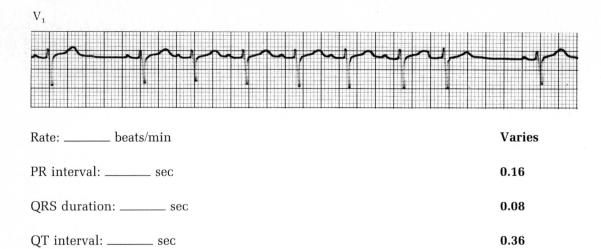

Rate: _____ beats/min   **Varies**

PR interval: _____ sec   **0.16**

QRS duration: _____ sec   **0.08**

QT interval: _____ sec   **0.36**

Conclusion: _____   **PSVT**

This paroxysmal supraventricular tachycardia (PSVT) is due to SA nodal reentry. This type of PSVT can begin with a sinus P wave or a premature atrial ectopic beat. The impulse enters the sinus node again and again in a reentry circuit to produce a tachycardia with sinus P waves. In this case the tachycardia is finally terminated by a PAC, seen distorting the T wave before the end of the tachycardia.

Tracing 1-15

II

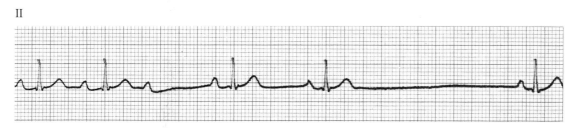

Rate: _____ beats/min   **Varies**

PR interval: _____ sec   **Varies**

QRS duration: _____ sec   **0.08**

QT interval: _____ sec   **Varies**

Conclusion: _____   **Sick sinus syndrome**

Sick sinus syndrome can take many forms. In this case the sinus node slows, there is an escape atrial beat, and then a pause of almost 2.5 sec without either a junctional or atrial escape beat, before the sinus node finally begins to beat.

The term "sick sinus syndrome" implies more than just sinus node dysfunction. There is also a failure of an adequate escape pacemaker, adversely influencing cerebral perfusion.

2

SUPRAVENTRICULAR ECTOPICS

- ☐ **Premature atrial complexes**
- ☐ **Atrial tachycardia**
- ☐ **Junctional beats**
- ☐ **Accelerated junctional rhythm**
- ☐ **Junctional tachycardia**
- ☐ **Paroxysmal supraventricular tachycardia**
- ☐ **Atrial flutter**
- ☐ **Atrial fibrillation**

Premature atrial complex

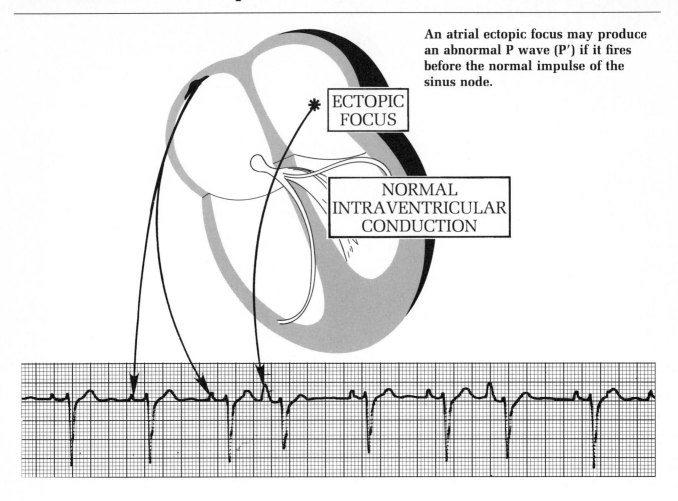

An atrial ectopic focus may produce an abnormal P wave (P′) if it fires before the normal impulse of the sinus node.

ECTOPIC FOCUS

NORMAL INTRAVENTRICULAR CONDUCTION

A premature atrial complex (PAC) has a different shape from the _____ _____ _____.

**sinus
P wave**

A PAC is the result of an atrial _____ focus.

ectopic

A PAC may be conducted through the AV node and be followed by a normal _____.

QRS

An _____ P wave is called P prime (P′).

ectopic

Nonconducted PAC

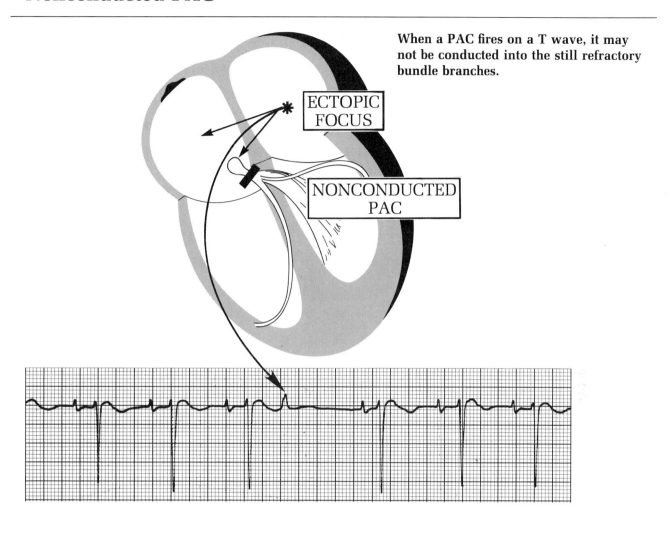

When a PAC fires on a T wave, it may not be conducted into the still refractory bundle branches.

ECTOPIC FOCUS

NONCONDUCTED PAC

Nonconducted PACs are very _____ in the cycle.   **early**

Conduction is not possible because the _____ _____ are   **bundle branches**
still refractory.

A PAC may be buried in a _____ wave.   **T**

A PAC will _____ a T wave.   **distort**

Atrial tachycardia with block

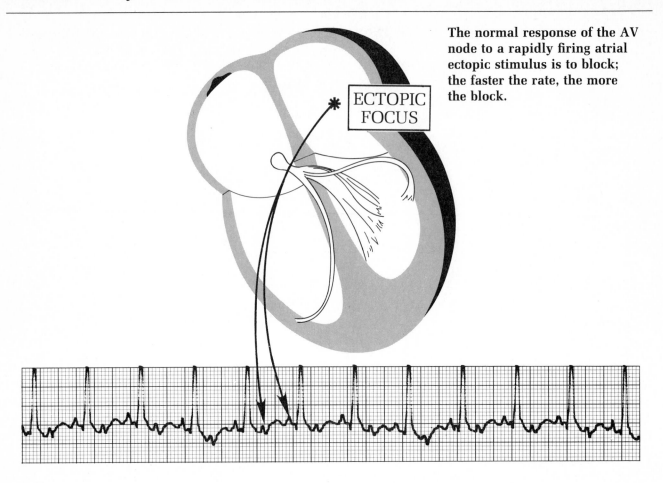

ECTOPIC FOCUS

The normal response of the AV node to a rapidly firing atrial ectopic stimulus is to block; the faster the rate, the more the block.

An atrial ectopic focus may fire repeatedly and dominate the heart. Intraventricular conduction may be _____.

normal

The rate of the atrial ectopic focus is _____ beats/min.

200

The ventricular rate is _____ beats/min.

100

The conduction ratio is _____.

2:1

Junctional beats

A junctional beat may be either premature or escape and may or may not be conducted up to the atria.

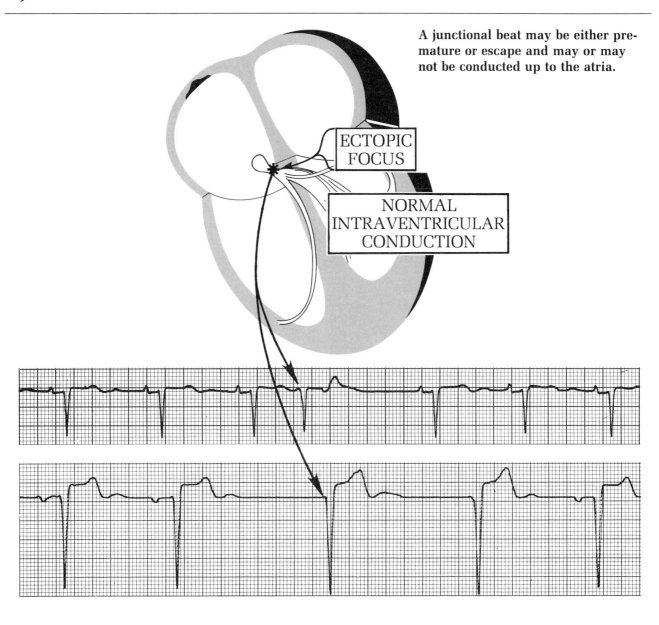

ECTOPIC FOCUS

NORMAL INTRAVENTRICULAR CONDUCTION

A junctional beat is recognized because the sinus _____ _____
is missing and ventricular conduction is _____.

P wave
normal

Junctional escape beats are a normal response to an abnormal condition;
premature junctional beats are _____ in themselves and often the
result of digitalis toxicity.

abnormal

Accelerated junctional rhythm

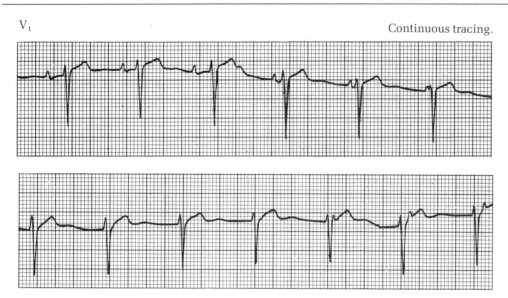

The inherent rate of the AV junction is 40 to 60 beats/min. Rates between 60 and 100 are considered accelerated. In a junctional rhythm or beat the P′ wave is sometimes not conducted retrogradely to the atria, leaving the sinus node in command of the atria (AV dissociation).

In this tracing the junctional rhythm begins to pace the ventricles at the _____ beat.   **fourth**

At the beginning of the tracing the rate of the sinus node is _____ beats/min.   **74**

The rate of the junctional focus is _____ beats/min.   **73**

The AV junction should not beat faster than 60 beats/min. Therefore this is an _____ _____ _____.   **accelerated junctional rhythm**

The ectopic focus in the junction manifests itself only because the sinus node _____.   **slows**

If the sinus rate had been faster, the junctional ectopic focus would have remained _____.   **hidden**

Junctional tachycardia

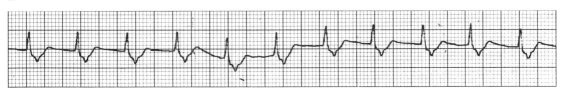

**When junctional rates exceed 100 beats/min, the term "tachycardia" is used.
In a junctional rhythm or beat the P' wave sometimes follows the QRS
complex; it may also occur just before or during the QRS complex.**

Each complex in this tracing is the result of a _____ ectopic beat.

junctional

The junctional ectopic focus in this tracing is beating at a rate of _____
beats/min.

110

Therefore this is a junctional _____.

tachycardia

If the rate of this rhythm had been below 100 beats/min, it would have been
called an _____ _____ _____.

**accelerated junctional
rhythm**

When the junction is beating at a rate greater than 60 beats/min,
_____ toxicity is often the cause.

digitalis

Junctional escape

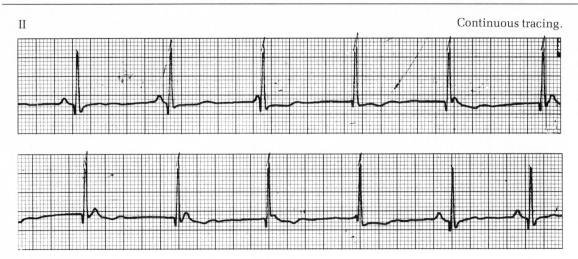

Sometimes a junctional rhythm is a normal escape mechanism, protecting the heart from excessively slow rates.

In this tracing the junctional rhythm begins to pace the ventricles at the _____ beat.

third

At the beginning of the tracing the rate of the sinus node is _____ beats/ min.

58

The rate of the junctional focus is _____ beats/min.

59

The normal rate of the AV junction is between 40 and 60 beats/min. Therefore this is a _____ _____ _____ _____.

normal junctional escape rhythm

The ectopic focus in the junction manifests itself only because the sinus node _____.

slows

Paroxysmal supraventricular tachycardia

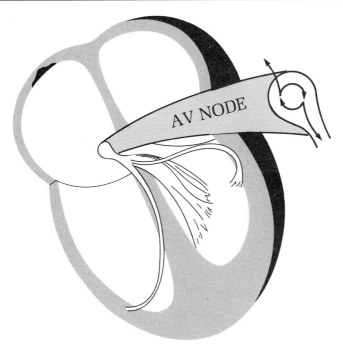

An AV nodal reentry mechanism is a common cause of paroxysmal supraventricular tachycardia (PSVT). The reentry circuit may begin with a single premature atrial, junctional, or ventricular beat.

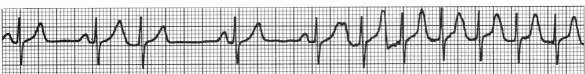

In this tracing the reentry circuit begins with a single _____.

PAC

A PAC enters the ventricles, using only part of the _____ _____.

AV node

The impulse then returns to the atria through the other part of the _____ _____.

AV node

Thus a _____ circuit is established.

reentry

This PSVT begins with _____ PAC and is supported by a _____ _____.

one; reentry circuit

Atrial flutter

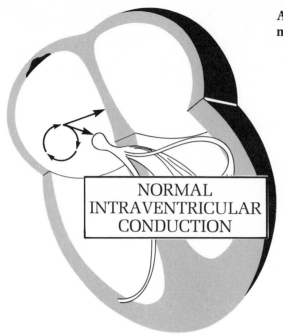

Atrial flutter is thought to be the result of a microreentry circuit within the atria.

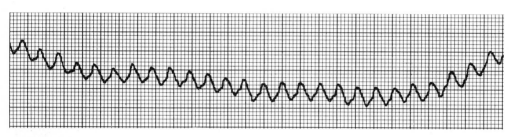

Atrial flutter has a typical sawtooth pattern.

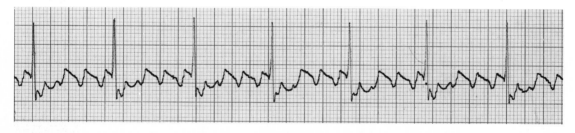

The sawtooth pattern of atrial flutter is distorted by ventricular complexes and T waves. The conduction ratio in atrial flutter is usually 2:1 or 4:1.

Atrial fibrillation

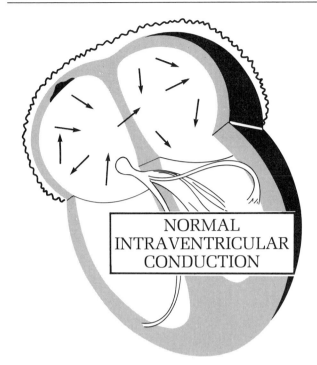

Atrial fibrillation results in many currents bombarding the AV node, some of which penetrate incompletely (concealed conduction), leaving the AV junction refractory and producing an irregular ventricular rhythm.

NORMAL INTRAVENTRICULAR CONDUCTION

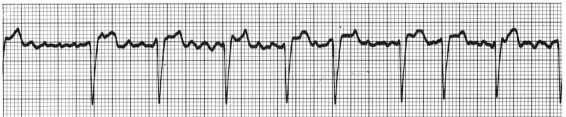

The ventricular rhythm is irregular in uncomplicated atrial fibrillation because of _____ _____. **concealed conduction**

When the atria are fibrillating they cannot _____. **contract**

There are no P waves in atrial fibrillation because the atria are _____. **fibrillating**

Tracing 2-1

II

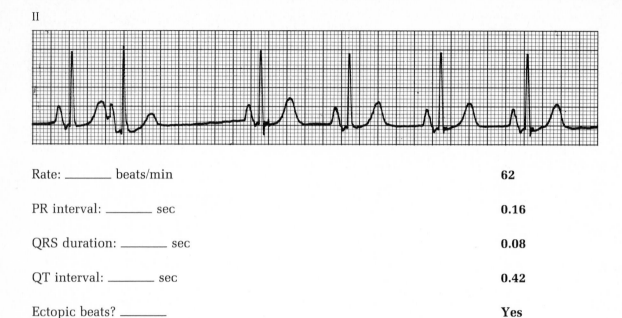

Rate: _____ beats/min	**62**
PR interval: _____ sec	**0.16**
QRS duration: _____ sec	**0.08**
QT interval: _____ sec	**0.42**
Ectopic beats? _____	**Yes**
What kind? _____	**Atrial**
Conclusion: _____	**PAC**

A PAC causes an irregularity in the underlying sinus rhythm. The P′ wave in this case is close to the preceding T wave. Sometimes a P′ wave that is this premature will not conduct at all because of the refractoriness of the ventricles or may be conducted abnormally for the same reason.

In this tracing we have opportunity to notice how heart rate will change the action potential duration. The QT interval after the long pause is 0.06 sec longer than the others.

In the setting of the coronary care unit the cause of frequent PACs should be investigated. They may be one of the first signs of congestive heart failure, since increased left-ventricular pressure would be reflected back to the atria, causing stretch of the atrial fibers and ectopic beats. Digitalis toxicity is also a consideration, as are hypoxia and acid-base imbalance.

Tracing 2-2

V$_1$

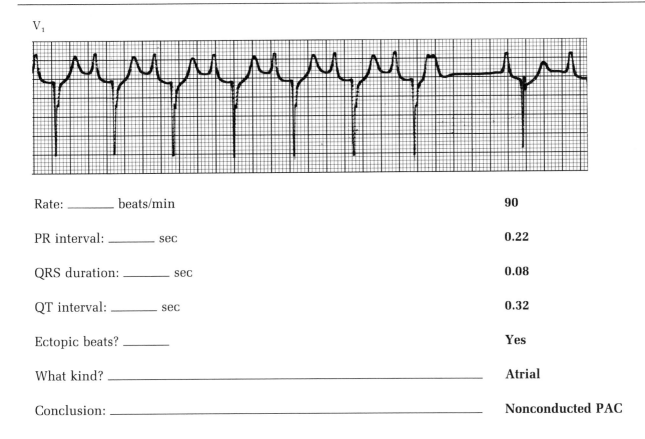

Rate: _____ beats/min	**90**
PR interval: _____ sec	**0.22**
QRS duration: _____ sec	**0.08**
QT interval: _____ sec	**0.32**
Ectopic beats? _____	**Yes**
What kind? _____	**Atrial**
Conclusion: _____	**Nonconducted PAC**

Here is the great imitator, the nonconducted PAC. This arrhythmia is commonly incorrectly called SA block or sinus arrest. Whenever you encounter an unexpected pause, remember that the nonconducted P' is far more common than SA block. Carefully examine the T wave preceding the pause and compare it with the other T waves in the tracing. They should all be the same shape. In this particular tracing the T wave before the pause has what appears to be an elevated ST segment. If you compare this T wave with the others, you will notice that the elevation is caused by a hidden P' wave.

There are two other features in this tracing that warrant your attention: first-degree heart block (long PR interval) and junctional escape beat. The heart block is discussed in detail in Chapter 4. You would have been unaware of the junctional escape beat unless you are very discerning. Notice (1) that the PR interval after the pause is shorter than the others because the latent pacemaker in the AV junction fired and captured the ventricles before the sinus beat had a chance to do so and (2) that the ventricular complex after the pause is slightly different from the others. The latter is a very helpful sign in locating the junctional escape beats. The slightly different shape occurs because sometimes the location of the junctional escape focus is a little offset within the AV junction.

Tracing 2-3

II

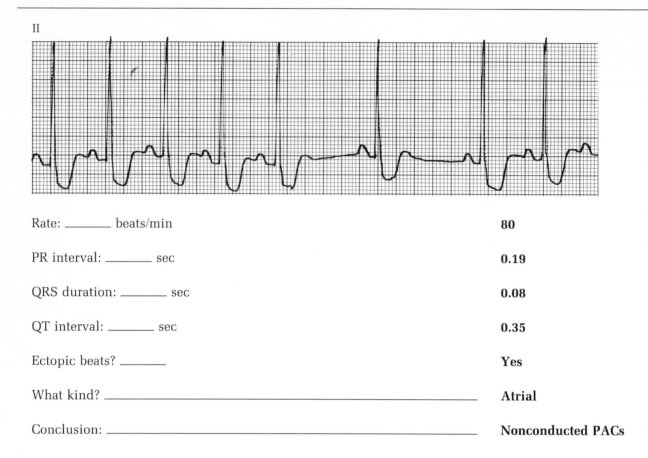

Rate: _____ beats/min **80**

PR interval: _____ sec **0.19**

QRS duration: _____ sec **0.08**

QT interval: _____ sec **0.35**

Ectopic beats? _____ **Yes**

What kind? _____ **Atrial**

Conclusion: _____ **Nonconducted PACs**

There are two nonconducted PACs in this tracing. When you encounter an unexpected pause, this should be the first thing you think of. If you compare the T waves before the pause with the others, you can easily see the distortion caused by the hidden P′ waves. Remember that all of the T waves should be the same shape.

Apart from distorting the T waves, the hidden P′ waves manifest their presence in another way. Notice that the sinus rhythm after the last pause begins somewhat slower than the sinus rhythm preceding the pauses. This phenomenon is called overdrive suppression. It is a property of all pacemaker cells and means that the inherent rate of a pacemaker cell may be suppressed when that cell is stimulated from another source. For example, when the sinus node cells are stimulated by an ectopic focus, often one or two cycles occur before the sinus rate is back to what it was before the intrusion.

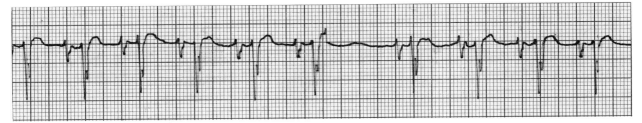

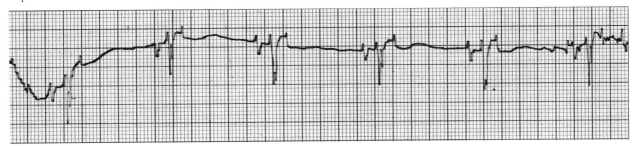

Bigeminal nonconducted PACs simulate the sudden onset of sinus bradycardia. In the top tracing above, there is one nonconducted PAC (in the T before the pause). PACs can also be seen distorting the T waves of the bottom tracing, which is from the same patient. Nonconducted PACs are more common than the conditions they mimic—namely, SA block and sinus arrest.

II

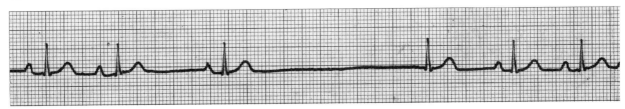

The tracing above is an example of sinus arrest. The third P wave is an atrial escape beat; there is a long pause and then a junctional escape beat before the sinus node finally beats again.

Tracing 2-4

Continuous tracing.

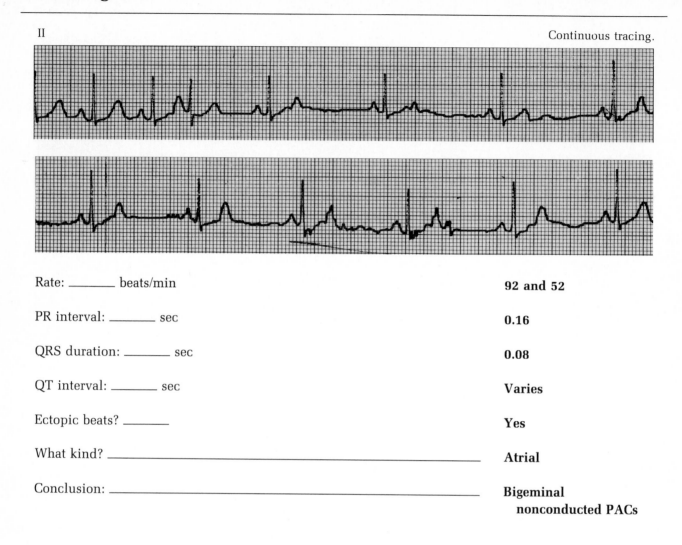

Rate: _____ beats/min	**92 and 52**
PR interval: _____ sec	**0.16**
QRS duration: _____ sec	**0.08**
QT interval: _____ sec	**Varies**
Ectopic beats? _____	**Yes**
What kind? _____	**Atrial**
Conclusion: _____	**Bigeminal nonconducted PACs**

Although somatic tremor distorts some of this tracing, it is evident that bigeminal nonconducted PACs simulate a sudden onset of sinus bradycardia. Because the treatment for sinus bradycardia and PACs is so completely different, it is important to make a differential diagnosis. The first PAC occurs after the second beat and is normally conducted. There is a nonconducted P' wave in the fourth T wave and in every T wave following. Remember that a PAC is not part of the T wave mechanism and so will distort the T a little differently each time.

If you remember the normal physiology of the sinus node and remember to compare T waves, the P' waves will be easily detected. The healthy sinus node does not suddenly jump into a sinus bradycardia or a sinus tachycardia. These arrhythmias ensue gradually in response to lessened or quickened body needs.

Tracing 2-5

MCL

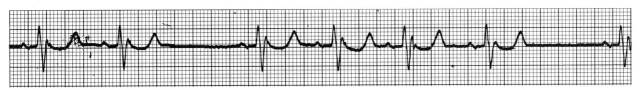

Rate: _____ beats/min   **Varies**

PR interval: _____ sec   **0.18**

QRS duration: _____ sec   **0.16**

QT interval: _____ sec   **Varies**

Ectopic beats? _____   **No**

What kind? _____   **Not applicable**

Conclusion: _____   **SA Wenckebach**

There are no P waves in the T waves preceding the pauses. This may be an atypical SA Wenckebach, since the PP interval shortens between the first cycle and the second cycle, starting with the P wave after the first pause.

Tracing 2-6

II

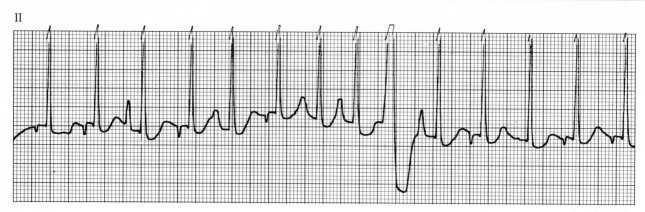

Rate: _____ beats/min

PR interval: _____ sec

QRS duration: _____ sec

QT interval: _____ sec

Ectopic beats? _____

What kind? _____

Conclusion: _____

_____

Varies

Ectopic P waves

0.08

Varies

Yes

Multifocal atrial

Multifocal PAC (chaotic atrial tachycardia)

Multifocal PACs are sometimes called chaotic atrial tachycardia. This arrhythmia is the one most commonly seen during acute respiratory failure.

At least four different P' wave shapes can be seen throughout the strip. The first three P' waves are all different in morphology from each other, and the third P' wave from the end is different still. These differences indicate that many ectopic foci are assuming pacemaker function in the atria.

42

Tracing 2-7

II

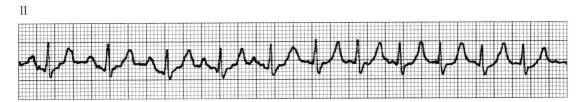

Rate: _____ beats/min   **92 (underlying)**

PR interval: _____ sec   **0.18**

QRS duration: _____ sec   **0.09**

QT interval: _____ sec   **0.32**

Ectopic beats? _____   **Yes**

What kind? _____   **Atrial**

Conclusion: _____   **PSVT**

This type of PSVT is sometimes called paroxysmal AV nodal tachycardia, reciprocating tachycardia, or AV nodal reentry tachycardia. It begins abruptly with a PAC (the fourth P wave), after which a reciprocating mechanism sustains the tachycardia. This means that the PAC has caused one part of the AV node to be out of phase with the other. That is, the impulse is conducted down one pathway and not the other. The ventricles are captured normally; however, the impulse can now pass retrogradely (backward) up the AV node through the nonrefractory pathway to depolarize the atria (atrial echo beat). By this time the other side of the AV node is nonrefractory, and the stimulus passes antegradely (forward) down the node to recapture the ventricle (a reciprocal beat). This circuit continues around and around in the AV node. It may be interrupted by a vagal maneuver or an appropriately timed stimulus. The atria may or may not be involved in the circuit. This is the most common mechanism of paroxysmal supraventricular tachycardia.

Tracing 2-8

II

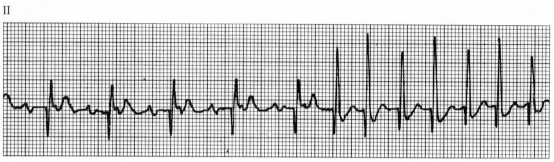

Rate: _____ beats/min

PR interval: _____ sec

QRS duration: _____ sec

QT interval: _____ sec

Ectopic beats? _____

What kind? _____

Conclusion: _____

_____

86 (underlying)

Ectopic P waves

0.08

0.32

Yes

Atrial

Atrial tachycardia with block followed by PSVT

In the first half of the tracing there is atrial tachycardia (an atrial ectopic focus) with 2:1 conduction. There are P′ waves distorting the ST segment. Most probably, one of the atrial ectopic stimuli was blocked in only one descending pathway, so that a retrograde pathway was created and an AV nodal reentry mechanism established.

Tracing 2-9

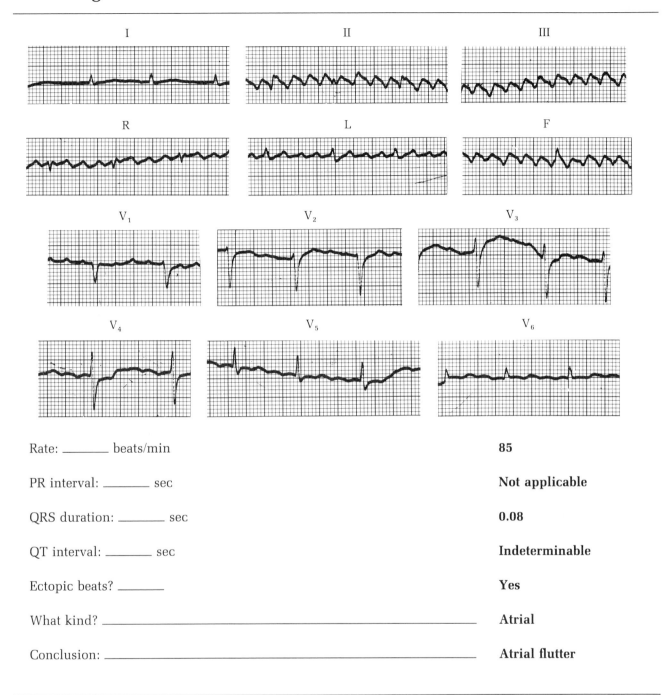

Rate: _____ beats/min   **85**

PR interval: _____ sec   **Not applicable**

QRS duration: _____ sec   **0.08**

QT interval: _____ sec   **Indeterminable**

Ectopic beats? _____   **Yes**

What kind? _____   **Atrial**

Conclusion: _____   **Atrial flutter**

This is atrial flutter with 4:1 conduction. Notice that in the inferior leads (II, III, and aV_F) the ventricular complex is barely detectable. This gives you an opportunity to notice the absolutely regular, uninterrupted cadence of the flutter waves. Notice that the P' waves are not seen at all in leads I, V₂, and V₃ in this particular patient, and yet atrial flutter is still present. In V₁ the P' waves are seen as little sharp peaks, much as a child would draw an ocean.

Tracing 2-10

II

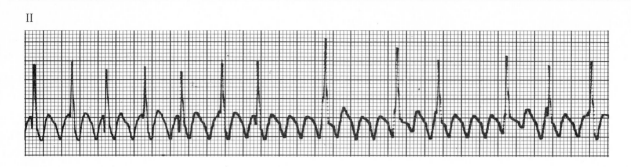

Rate: _____ beats/min   **Varies**

PR interval: _____ sec   **Not applicable**

QRS duration: _____ sec   **0.09**

QT interval: _____ sec   **0.32**

Ectopic beats? _____   **Yes**

What kind? _____   **Atrial**

Conclusion: _____   **Atrial flutter with**
                                                         variable AV
_____   **conduction**

The typical sawtooth pattern of atrial flutter is unmistakable in this tracing. The atrial rate is 300 beats/min, with variable block. In the beginning of the tracing the conduction ratio is 2:1, giving way to 4:1 and going back to 2:1.

This arrhythmia is thought to be the result of a reentry mechanism within the atria. It begins with one appropriately timed PAC and is easily terminated by cardioversion.

Notice that the P′ waves are right on time, with no pause to wait for the ventricular response. Atrial flutter is usually very easily spotted in the inferior leads (II, III, and aV$_F$) because of its typical distinguishing morphology. In these leads the P′ waves are the negative component and the Ta wave (atrial repolarization wave) is the positive component of the sawtooth pattern. In V$_1$ small upright P′ waves are usually seen. The 12-lead ECG on p. 47 illustrates the changing faces of atrial flutter in the different leads. Notice V$_3$ and compare it with aV$_F$. There is 2:1 AV conduction, which is easily seen in the inferior lead (aV$_F$) but is completely camouflaged in V$_3$. Sometimes, even in lead II, a 2:1 conduction is missed because one of the flutter waves is hidden in the QRS complex and the T wave.

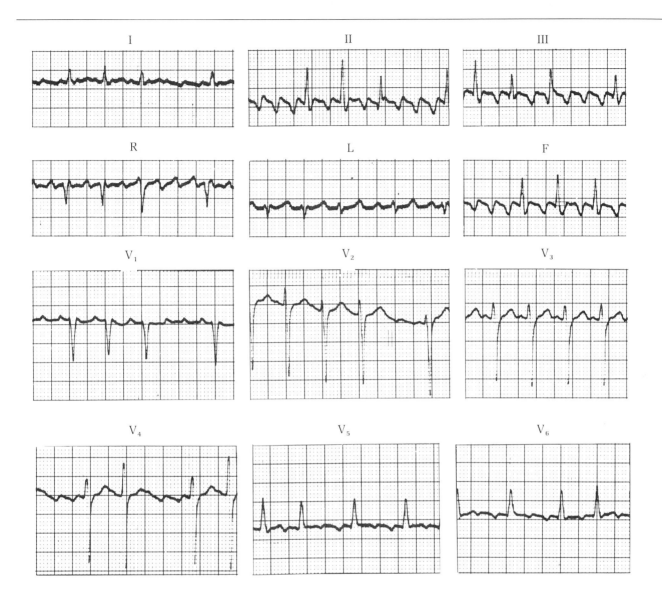

Tracing 2-11

V₁

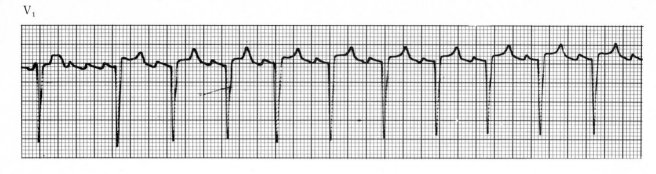

Rate: _____ beats/min	**100**
PR interval: _____ sec	**Not applicable**
QRS duration: _____ sec	**0.08**
QT interval: _____ sec	**Indeterminable**
Ectopic beats? _____	**Yes**
What kind? _____	**Atrial**
Conclusion: _____ _____	**Atrial flutter with variable AV conduction**

This is an atrial flutter with an atrial rate of 300 beats/min and varying AV conduction ratio. At the onset of the tracing the conduction ratio is 4:1. After that it is 3:1, a rare conduction ratio in atrial flutter. Sometimes in atrial flutter when the conduction ratio is 2:1 or 3:1, the QRS-T will hide the flutter waves.

It is usually necessary to walk out the P′ waves in order to determine the conduction ratio. Three P′ waves in a row are easily seen at the beginning of the tracing. Place a piece of paper under these and mark them off. Then move the paper and mark the same ones again until you have about six or seven evenly spaced marks on your paper. Now place these marks across the ventricular complexes, with the first mark on the P′ wave preceding the QRS. You will see that there are three P′ waves for every QRS. It is easy to see that if only the last part of the tracing, and only lead V₁, were available to you, you probably would not have diagnosed atrial flutter.

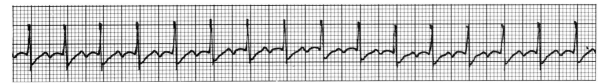

Atrial flutter with 2:1 AV conduction.

In the figure above the conduction ratio is 2:1. It is a good rule to always suspect atrial flutter when the heart rate is around 150, as it is here.

Tracing 2-12

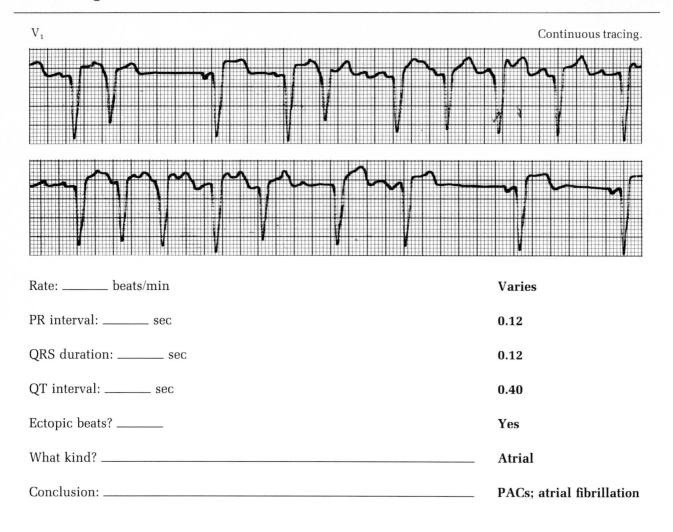

Rate: _____ beats/min   **Varies**

PR interval: _____ sec   **0.12**

QRS duration: _____ sec   **0.12**

QT interval: _____ sec   **0.40**

Ectopic beats? _____   **Yes**

What kind? _____   **Atrial**

Conclusion: _____   **PACs; atrial fibrillation**

This patient has frequent PACs, which eventually produce a paroxysm of atrial fibrillation. The tracing begins with two PACs, followed by a normal sinus beat and two more PACs. This time the second P′ in the group produces atrial fibrillation. A short P-P′ interval results in electrical disunity in the atria and atrial fibrillation. In the second strip the arrhythmia is seen to convert spontaneously into a sinus rhythm.

The patient's main electrocardiographic problem is that of sinus bradycardia and PACs. In this case the atrial fibrillation is a result of the PACs. A paroxysm of atrial fibrillation causes a sudden fall in both cardiac output and coronary perfusion. It is, therefore, important to protect this patient from further bouts of atrial fibrillation. It is necessary to ensure adequate oxygenation. The electrolyte panel should be checked, and a third heart sound should be listened for, since PACs are also an early sign of congestive heart failure.

Tracing 2-13

V_1

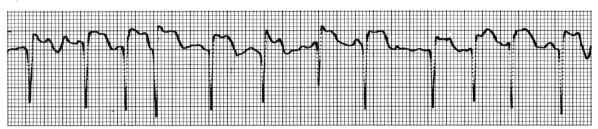

Rate: _____ beats/min   **Varies**

PR interval: _____ sec   **Not applicable**

QRS duration: _____ sec   **0.06**

QT interval: _____ sec   **Varies**

Ectopic beats? _____   **Yes**

What kind? _____   **Atrial**

Conclusion: _____   **Atrial fibrillation**

The grossly irregular ventricular rhythm is what you would expect in this arrhythmia. The rate indicates that it is uncontrolled (not adequately treated).

One of a number of drugs may be used to slow the ventricular rate. Digitalis lengthens the refractory period at the AV node, limiting the number of impulses that can penetrate. Since there is no PR interval to gauge the effect of the digitalis on AV conduction, you must pay special attention to any regularization of the ventricular rhythm and to the noncardiac symptoms of digitalis toxicity. Remember that in atrial fibrillation the ventricular response *should* be absolutely irregular. If heart block is present, a junctional pacemaker will pace the ventricles. This pacemaker will be protected from the chaotic activity in the atria by the block, which may be either complete or intermittent. The ventricular rhythm will then be absolutely regular, or intermittent regularity will be seen in the case of incomplete block. Digitalis, if given in excess, will cause heart block and may also result in an accelerated junctional rhythm or junctional tachycardia.

Tracing 2-14

V₁

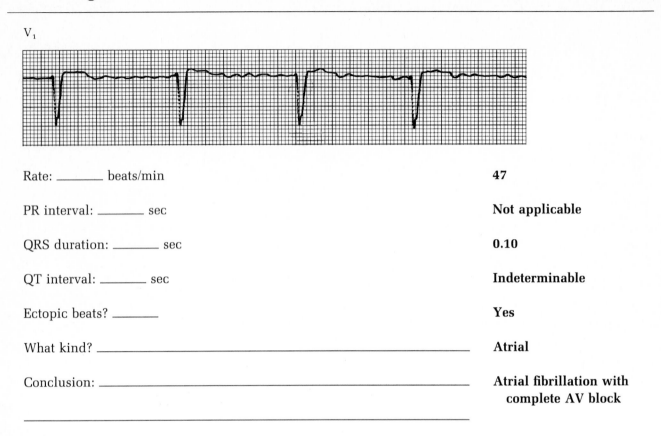

Rate: _____ beats/min   **47**

PR interval: _____ sec   **Not applicable**

QRS duration: _____ sec   **0.10**

QT interval: _____ sec   **Indeterminable**

Ectopic beats? _____   **Yes**

What kind? _____   **Atrial**

Conclusion: _____   **Atrial fibrillation with
                                                    complete AV block**

The fibrillatory line is clearly seen through the tracing. However, the ventricular rhythm is absolutely regular at approximately 47 beats/min. This indicates complete heart block. This patient has not received digitalis; therefore, it is a pathological block and is not drug induced.

Tracing 2-15

V₁

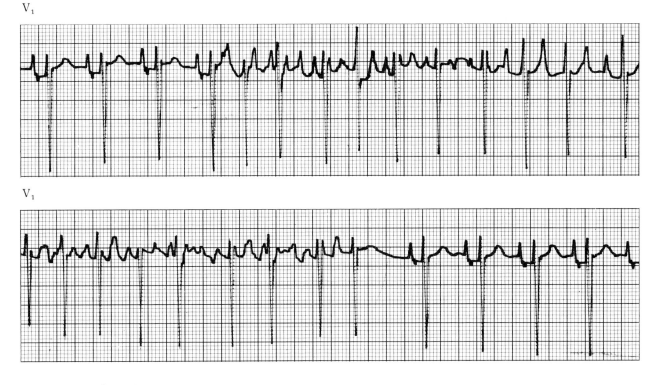

V₁

Rate: _____ beats/min	**100-140**
PR interval: _____ sec	**0.15**
QRS duration: _____ sec	**0.08**
QT interval: _____ sec	**0.32**
Ectopic beats? _____	**Yes**
What kind? _____	**Atrial**
Conclusion: _____	**Atrial flutter-fibrillation**

In this tracing atrial flutter-fibrillation has resulted from a very short P-P' interval. The beginning of the tracing is a sinus rhythm of 100. The first P' wave is easily seen distorting the fourth T wave. The second tracing, which is from the same patient, shows spontaneous conversion into a sinus rhythm.

The hemodynamic consequences of a sudden onset of atrial fibrillation for the myocardial infarct patient can be very serious. Fibrillating atria do not pump blood. The atrial kick accounts for 20% of the cardiac output, a loss that an ischemic myocardium cannot afford.

Tracing 2-16

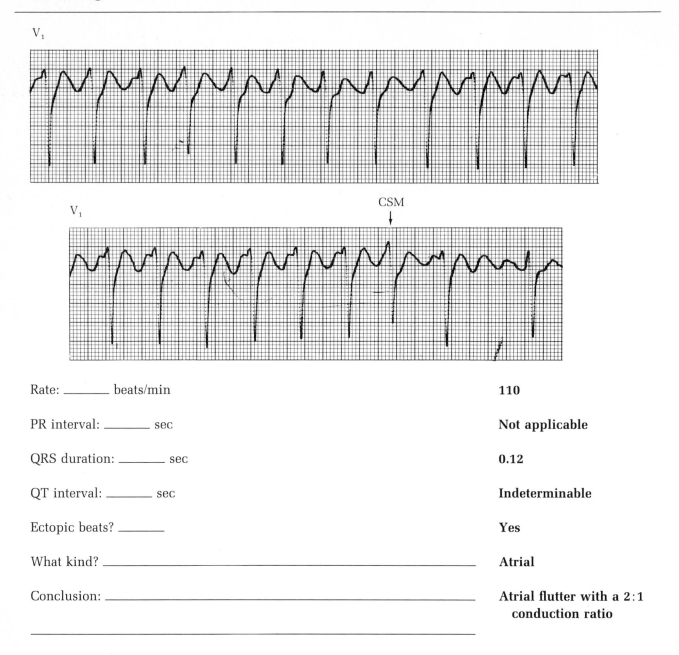

V₁

CSM

V₁

Rate: _____ beats/min   **110**

PR interval: _____ sec   **Not applicable**

QRS duration: _____ sec   **0.12**

QT interval: _____ sec   **Indeterminable**

Ectopic beats? _____   **Yes**

What kind? _____   **Atrial**

Conclusion: _____   **Atrial flutter with a 2:1**
                                                               conduction ratio

In the first tracing there are no distinct P waves. The changing bulge in front of the r waves should cause you to suspect the hidden flutter wave (atrial flutter with 2:1 block). This diagnosis is confirmed in the second tracing, from the same patient, where a 4:1 conduction ratio is seen in response to carotid sinus massage (CSM). Clearly seen at the end of the tracing is the undulating pattern of atrial flutter. However, the atrial rate is only 220 to 224 beats/min. Some authorities would call this an atrial tachycardia and say that it would be an atrial flutter only if the atrial rate exceeded 250 beats/min. Others would say that no matter what the rate, a sawtooth pattern is atrial flutter. Regardless of what this condition is called, the main consideration is that a rapid ventricular rate has resulted from an ectopic atrial tachycardia.

Tracing 2-17

II

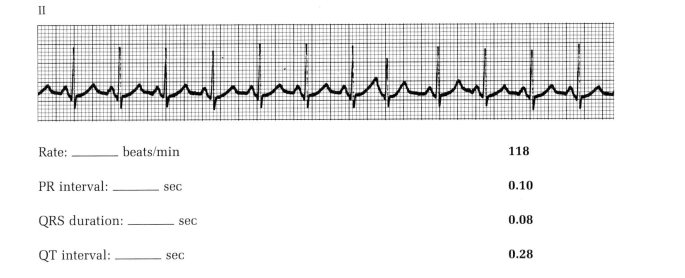

Rate: _____ beats/min   **118**

PR interval: _____ sec   **0.10**

QRS duration: _____ sec   **0.08**

QT interval: _____ sec   **0.28**

Ectopic beats? _____   **Yes**

What kind? _____   **Atrial**

Conclusion: _____   **Sinus tachycardia; PAC**

The single irregularity in this sinus tachycardia is caused by a PAC. This P′ wave is hidden in a T wave in approximately the middle of the strip. It causes the T wave to be tall and peaked.

Sinus tachycardia in a resting patient and PACs are both signs of congestive heart failure. They are not conclusive signs but should make you aware of a possible problem.

Tracing 2-18

V₁

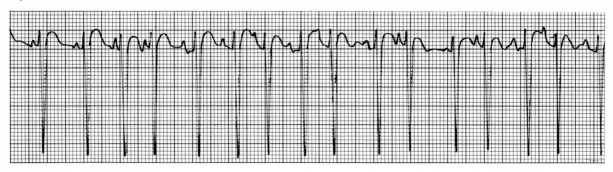

Rate: _____ beats/min   **140-160**

PR interval: _____ sec   **Ectopic P waves**

QRS duration: _____ sec   **0.08**

QT interval: _____ sec   **0.25**

Ectopic beats? _____   **Yes**

What kind? _____   **Atrial**

Conclusion: _____   **Chaotic atrial
                                                                 tachycardia**

This tracing represents chaotic atrial tachycardia, also known as multi-focal PACs. Because there are so many ectopic P waves (P′ waves), it is difficult to tell if there are any sinus P waves at all. This arrhythmia is said to often accompany pulmonary disease and electrolyte imbalance.

Tracing 2-19

V₁

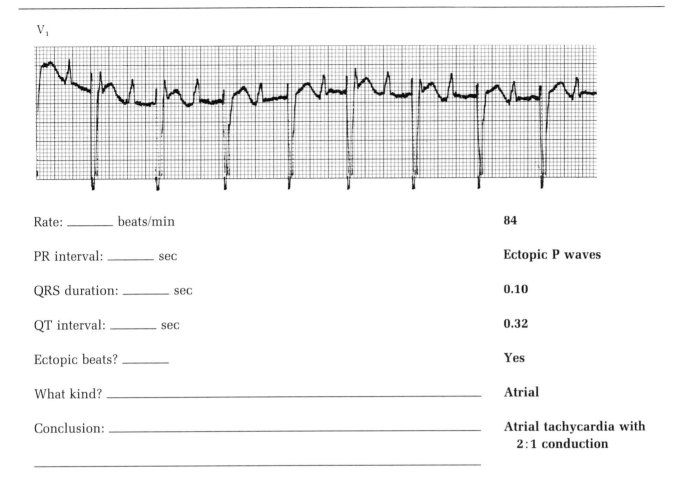

Rate: _____ beats/min	**84**
PR interval: _____ sec	**Ectopic P waves**
QRS duration: _____ sec	**0.10**
QT interval: _____ sec	**0.32**
Ectopic beats? _____	**Yes**
What kind? _____	**Atrial**
Conclusion: _____	**Atrial tachycardia with 2:1 conduction**

A slight somatic tremor runs through the tracing, but it is not enough to preclude a diagnosis of atrial tachycardia with 2:1 AV conduction. Notice that some of the ventricular complexes have an R′ wave, whereas others do not. That "R′" wave is really a P′ partially hidden by the ventricular complex. If you happened to use the QRS with this distortion to measure your QRS duration, you would have an incorrect and abnormally long measurement.

Whenever P waves are midway between two R waves, it is wise to always suspect a hidden P, which is the case here. If the hidden P had not been noticed, a diagnosis of first-degree heart block would have been made, when the patient really has an atrial tachycardia of 168 beats/min with 2:1 A-V conduction. This arrhythmia suggests a mechanism of enhanced automaticity in the atrium.

Tracing 2-20

II

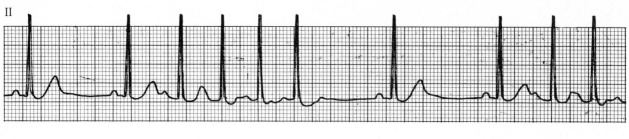

Rate: _____ beats/min   **56 (underlying)**

PR interval: _____ sec   **0.16**

QRS duration: _____ sec   **0.06**

QT interval: _____ sec   **0.40**

Ectopic beats? _____   **Yes**

What kind? _____   **Atrial**

Conclusion: _____   **PSVT**

The underlying rhythm is a sinus bradycardia of 56 beats/min. The supraventricular tachycardia begins with a PAC after the second R wave. It terminates and then begins again after two more sinus beats. This arrhythmia is an AV nodal reentry mechanism. It usually requires no treatment, is self-limiting, and can be terminated by a vagal maneuver. However, in a patient with myocardial infarction the tachycardia may further compromise coronary circulation.

Tracing 2-21

II

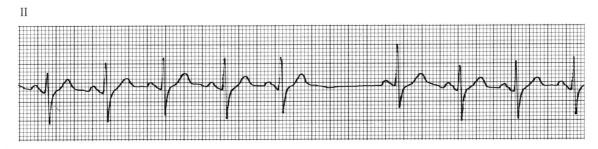

Rate: _____ beats/min	**92 (underlying)**
PR interval: _____ sec	**0.14**
QRS duration: _____ sec	**0.08**
QT interval: _____ sec	**0.32**
Ectopic beats? _____	**Yes**
What kind? _____	**Atrial**
Conclusion: _____	**Nonconducted PAC**

There is probably a nonconducted PAC in this tracing. The T wave preceding the pause is only slightly distorted. However, there is a slowing of the sinus rhythm after the pause. A PAC would cause such a suppression. Also, SA block is far less frequent. Statistics alone would favor the nonconducted PAC.

In this tracing you have another opportunity to notice how the length of the refractory period changes with heart rate. Notice the difference between the QT interval preceding the pause and that of the one following it. As the length of the cycle increases, the refractory period also increases.

Tracing 2-22

V_1

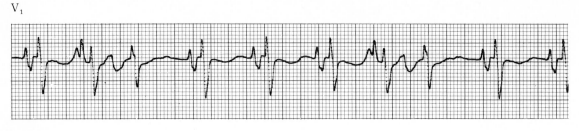

Rate: _____ beats/min	**84**
PR interval: _____ sec	**0.16**
QRS duration: _____ sec	**0.10**
QT interval: _____ sec	**0.38**
Ectopic beats? _____	**Yes**
What kind? _____	**Atrial**
Conclusion: _____	**PSVT**

The irregularity in this tracing is due to PACs followed by a reciprocating mechanism. Two PACs are very apparent; they precede the second and the seventh beats and are normally conducted. Notice the T wave following the first PAC of each group. It is distorted with a P′ wave and followed by a normal ventricular complex. The first PAC was conducted into the ventricles via a slow AV nodal pathway, and activated the ventricles normally while at the same time returning to the atria via a previously blocked fast pathway. Once the impulse is in the atria the anterograde slow pathway becomes available and the impulse descends into the ventricles to once again activate them. Then the mechanism stops, at least for the moment. This reciprocating mechanism later continued for this patient, producing a supraventricular tachycardia.

A reciprocating mechanism consisting of only two or three beats should serve to warn of the possibility of a sustained AV nodal reentry and a perhaps debilitating tachycardia for the patient who has myocardial infarction. Every effort should be made to discover and treat the cause of the PAC so that a reciprocating mechanism will not be initiated.

Tracing 2-23

V₁

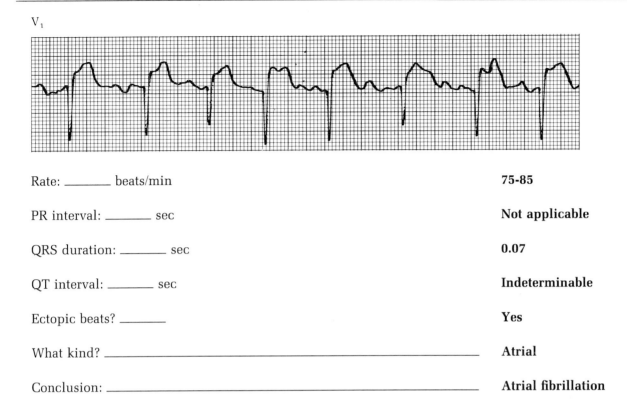

Rate: _____ beats/min	**75-85**
PR interval: _____ sec	**Not applicable**
QRS duration: _____ sec	**0.07**
QT interval: _____ sec	**Indeterminable**
Ectopic beats? _____	**Yes**
What kind? _____	**Atrial**
Conclusion: _____	**Atrial fibrillation**

This atrial fibrillation is said to be "controlled" because the ventricular rate has been slowed by a drug that lengthens the refractory period of the AV node—in this case, digitalis.

When digitalis toxicity is present during atrial fibrillation, the usual early ECG signs of digitalis toxicity (that is, premature junctional beats and first-degree AV block) do not show themselves. This is because during atrial fibrillation it is impossible to tell when there is an isolated junctional beat, and there are no P waves, so that AV conduction is severely impaired before toxicity is manifested. Thus the ECG signs of toxicity are late ones—enhanced automaticity in the AV junction and/or advanced block at the AV node. Either or both of these conditions during atrial fibrillation cause some or total regularization of the rhythm. Such a sign is seen in this tracing. Note that the second, fourth, and fifth cycle lengths are exactly the same and reveal an accelerated junctional rate of 75 beats/min. There may be some heart block present, but that cannot be known. We do know, however, that complete AV block is not present, since this would bar all atrial stimuli from penetrating into the bundle of His and would result in an absolutely regular junctional rhythm—not the case here. There is one exception to this: when the accelerated junctional focus is conducted to the ventricles in a Wenchebach fashion the ventricular complexes will be in groups, either pairs or groups of three or four.

Tracing 2-24

II

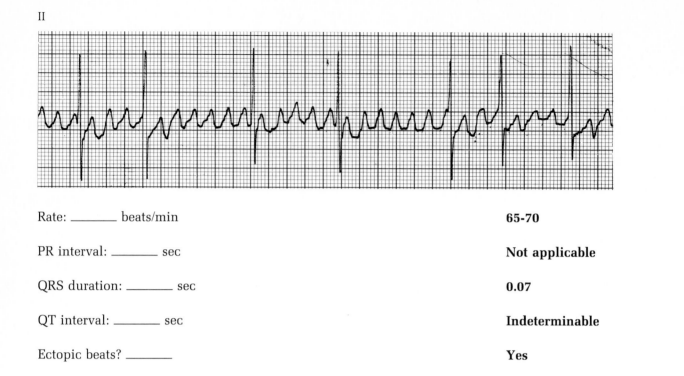

Rate: _____ beats/min

PR interval: _____ sec

QRS duration: _____ sec

QT interval: _____ sec

Ectopic beats? _____

What kind? _____

Conclusion: _____

_____

65-70

Not applicable

0.07

Indeterminable

Yes

Atrial

**Atrial flutter with
variable AV
conduction**

The atrial rate here is 300 beats/min, with anywhere from two to seven P waves for every QRS complex. With a 7:1 conduction ratio, some degree of pathological AV block would be suspected.

Tracing 2-25

II

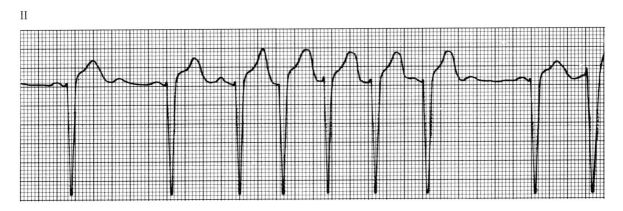

Rate: _____ beats/min   **55 (underlying)**

PR interval: _____ sec   **0.14**

QRS duration: _____ sec   **0.12**

QT interval: _____ sec   **0.42**

Ectopic beats? _____   **Yes**

What kind? _____   **Atrial**

Conclusion: _____   **PSVT**

Here again is an example of PSVT. The tracing begins with two sinus P waves. A prominent U wave is present. This is usually a sign of hypokalemia, which may have caused the PACs. A PAC follows the second complex, and a paroxysm of supraventricular tachycardia ensues. It terminates spontaneously.

Tracing 2-26

II

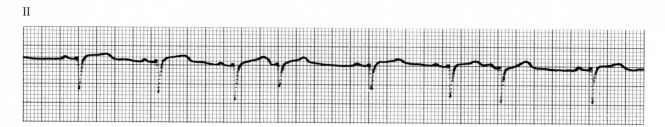

Rate: _____ beats/min   **70 (underlying)**

PR interval: _____ sec   **0.14**

QRS duration: _____ sec   **0.08**

QT interval: _____ sec   **0.38**

Ectopic beats? _____   **Yes**

What kind? _____   **Atrial**

Conclusion: _____   **PACs**

The irregularity in the above rhythm is caused by PACs occurring after the third and sixth beats. The first P′ wave is buried in a T wave and distorts it. The second P′ wave falls after a T wave, looking almost like a U wave.

Tracing 2-27

V₁

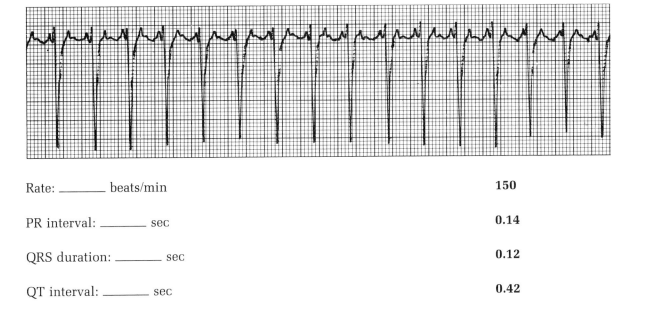

Rate: _____ beats/min	**150**
PR interval: _____ sec	**0.14**
QRS duration: _____ sec	**0.12**
QT interval: _____ sec	**0.42**
Ectopic beats? _____	**Yes**
What kind? _____	**Atrial**
Conclusion: _____	**Atrial flutter with 2:1 AV conduction**

There are two P′ waves for every QRS complex. The atrial rate is 300 beats/min. In lead II you would see the sawtooth pattern of atrial flutter, which often goes undetected when the conduction ratio is 2:1, as it is here. In lead V₁ above, the P′ waves are easily seen just before the ventricular complex and in the ST segment.

The AV conduction time is prolonged in atrial flutter because of concealed conduction. Very often it is as long as 0.46 sec, and it is seldom shorter than 0.24 sec. Note in this tracing that it is not the P′ wave immediately preceding the QRS that is conducted to the ventricles, but the one immediately following it.

Tracing 2-28

II

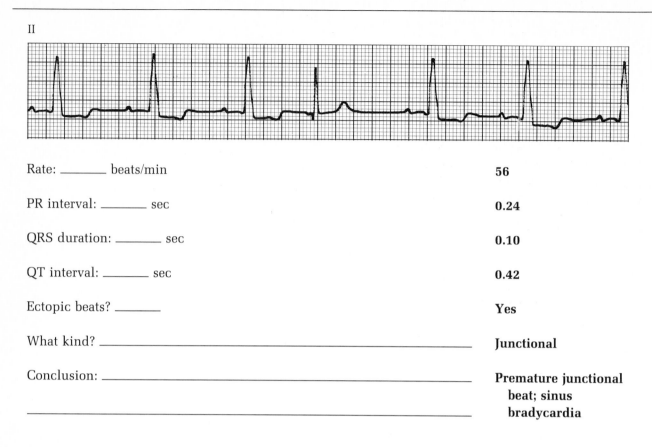

Rate: _____ beats/min	**56**
PR interval: _____ sec	**0.24**
QRS duration: _____ sec	**0.10**
QT interval: _____ sec	**0.42**
Ectopic beats? _____	**Yes**
What kind? _____	**Junctional**
Conclusion: _____	**Premature junctional beat; sinus bradycardia**

There is one beat in this tracing that causes the rhythm to be irregular. It is a premature junctional beat. Notice that it has a different shape from the sinus-conducted beats. Often a junctional beat is slightly different in shape because the focus is a little offset within the AV junction, causing its wave front to differ from that of a sinus-conducted beat. In the tracing above there may be another reason. Note that the junctional beat is narrower by 0.02 sec than the sinus beats. It may be that the broader QRS of the sinus beats is due to a small lesion in the bundle of His, rather than in the bundle branches, and that the junctional focus is below this lesion, producing normal conduction.

It is a matter of interest and not clinically important whether or not a junctional ectopic focus has conducted retrogradely to the atria. In the past the location of the P′ wave before, during, or after the ventricular complex was stressed. This is because it was thought that such information was an indicator of the precise site of the ectopic focus. It is now known that the location of the P′ wave is also a function of conduction velocity and therefore does not determine location.

In this tracing there is retrograde conduction to the atria, evidenced by the P′ wave in front of the junctional ectopic beat (P′-R interval: 0.06 sec). You will notice that there is a less than full compensatory pause. This in itself indicates premature firing of the sinus node from an ectopic focus.

Sinus bradycardia and first-degree heart block are also noted in this tracing. The latter diagnosis is made by measuring the PR interval and finding it to be greater than 0.20 sec. This is discussed more fully in Chapter 4.

Tracing 2-29

II

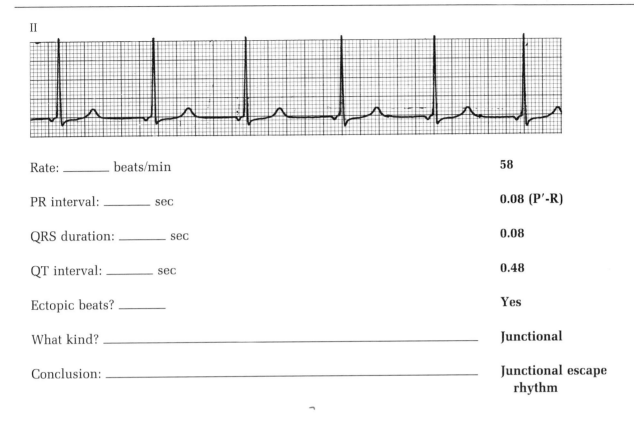

Rate: _____ beats/min	**58**
PR interval: _____ sec	**0.08 (P′-R)**
QRS duration: _____ sec	**0.08**
QT interval: _____ sec	**0.48**
Ectopic beats? _____	**Yes**
What kind? _____	**Junctional**
Conclusion: _____	**Junctional escape rhythm**

In lead II a negative P′ wave and a short P′-R interval (less than 0.12 sec) are two indicators of an ectopic junctional pacemaker. The P′-R interval in this case is 0.08 sec, and the ventricular complexes are clearly supraventricular. The rate is compatible with the inherent rate of the AV junctional pacemaker cells, qualifying this as a passive escape mechanism as opposed to an accelerated junctional rhythm. The pacemaker cells in the AV junction will usually escape and pace the heart if the sinus node fails to do so.

The treatment of this arrhythmia will depend on the hemodynamic state of the patient. The junctional escape rhythm itself will not be treated. If the patient is hypotensive, it may be necessary to increase the rate of the sinus node with atropine.

Tracing 2-30

II

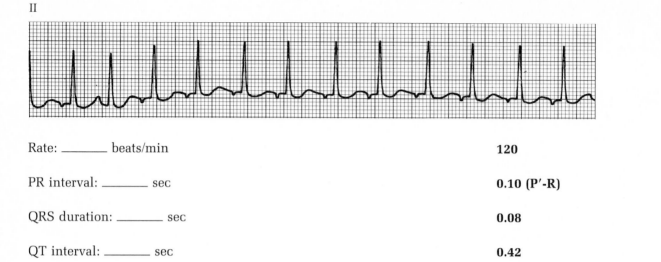

Rate: _____ beats/min

120

PR interval: _____ sec

0.10 (P′-R)

QRS duration: _____ sec

0.08

QT interval: _____ sec

0.42

Ectopic beats? _____

Yes

What kind? _____

Junctional

Conclusion: _____

Junctional tachycardia

Junctional tachycardia usually manifests with a rate of 70 to 130 beats/min and is commonly the result of digitalis excess. The slight irregularity in the tracing is the result of sinus capture (second beat, PR interval: 0.13 sec) or another ectopic focus.

This arrhythmia is thought to be the result of enhanced automaticity in the AV junction as opposed to the reentry mechanism seen in paroxysmal supraventricular tachycardia.

Tracing 2-31

V_1

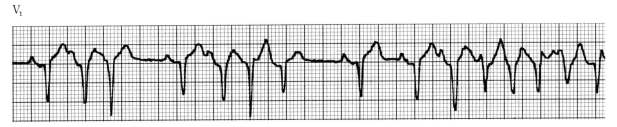

Rate: _____ beats/min   **100 (underlying)**

PR interval: _____ sec   **0.16**

QRS duration: _____ sec   **0.08**

QT interval: _____ sec   **0.26**

Ectopic beats? _____   **Yes**

What kind? _____   **Atrial**

Conclusion: _____   **PACs and PSVT**

This tracing shows bursts of PSVT, which are the result of very early PACs. There are three sinus P waves—one at the beginning of the tracing, one after the first pause, and two following the second pause. There is some somatic tremor artifact, which is probably the cause of the distortion of the fourth P wave. The two P waves in a row (middle of the tracing) allow us to note that the underlying sinus rhythm is 100 beats/min. This, along with the frequent PACs, should prompt a full physical assessment of the patient.

Tracing 2-32

V_1 Continuous tracing.

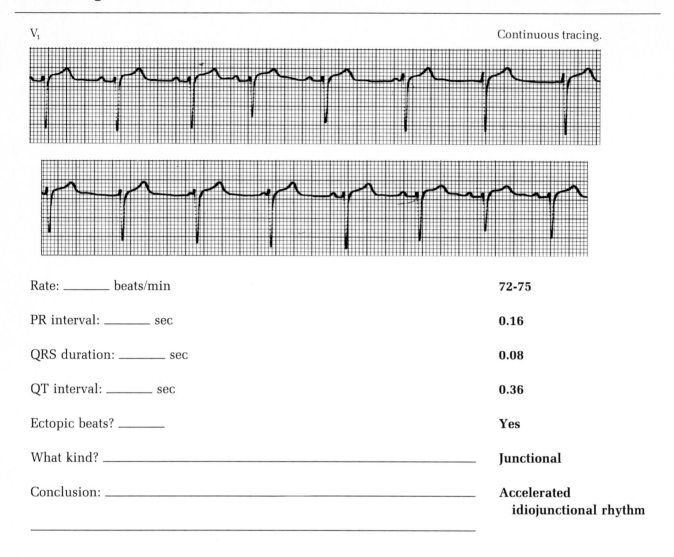

Rate: _____ beats/min   **72-75**

PR interval: _____ sec   **0.16**

QRS duration: _____ sec   **0.08**

QT interval: _____ sec   **0.36**

Ectopic beats? _____   **Yes**

What kind? _____   **Junctional**

Conclusion: _____   **Accelerated**
                                                               idiojunctional rhythm

_____

This is an accelerated idiojunctional rhythm at a rate of 73 beats/min, resulting in AV dissociation. There is an underlying sinus rhythm of 75 beats/min at the onset of the tracing. This slows to approximately 62, allowing the accelerated junctional focus to manifest itself.

One of the characteristics of latent pacemakers can be observed in this tracing. Latent pacemakers are normally suppressed by the sinus node. However, once they dominate and start beating, their rate increases slightly as they "warm up." In this case there is a sinus arrhythmia and when the sinus node slows down to 62 beats/min, the junctional focus takes over at an enhanced rate of 68, which increases to 72. The sinus rhythm finally increases its rate to 80 and reestablishes control, once again masking the existence of the accelerated junctional focus. This increase in sinus rate is probably an autonomic reflex occurring in response to the drop in blood pressure resulting from the AV dissociation.

Tracing 2-33

II

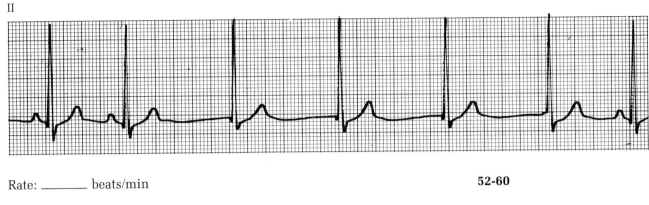

Rate: _____ beats/min

PR interval: _____ sec

QRS duration: _____ sec

QT interval: _____ sec

Ectopic beats? _____

What kind? _____

Conclusion: _____

52-60

0.16

0.10

0.40

Yes

Junctional

**Sinus arrest with
junctional escape**

This junctional escape mechanism is the result of an abrupt slowing or cessation of the sinus node impulse. When the sinus impulse fails to arrive at the AV junction, these pacemaker cells protect the ventricles at a normal escape rate (in this case, 52 beats/min). In the fourth junctional escape beat (sixth complex) the sinus P wave can be seen distorting the q wave.

Tracing 2-34

II

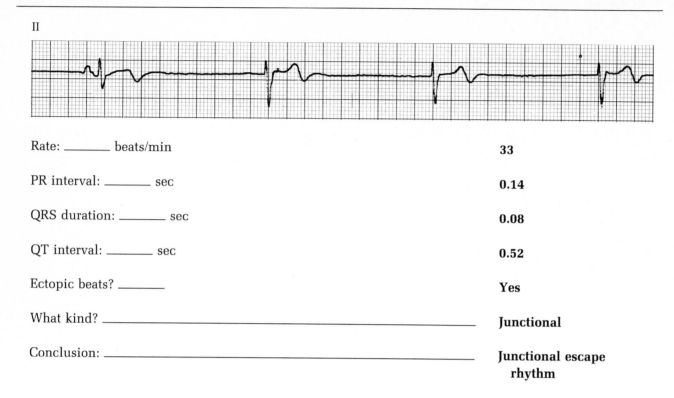

Rate: _____ beats/min   33

PR interval: _____ sec   0.14

QRS duration: _____ sec   0.08

QT interval: _____ sec   0.52

Ectopic beats? _____   Yes

What kind? _____   Junctional

Conclusion: _____   Junctional escape
                                                           rhythm

---

   The junctional escape rhythm in this tracing is the result of a profound
sinus bradycardia and sinus arrhythmia. The first beat is sinus conducted.
Note the differing morphology between the junctional escape beat and the
sinus-conducted one (Tracing 2-28). The hemodynamic impact of this profound bradycardia will determine the treatment.

Tracing 2-35

II

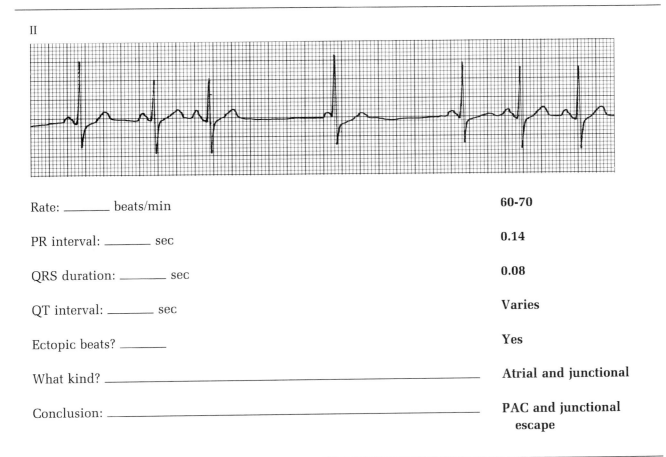

Rate: _____ beats/min

PR interval: _____ sec

QRS duration: _____ sec

QT interval: _____ sec

Ectopic beats? _____

What kind? _____

Conclusion: _____

60-70

0.14

0.08

Varies

Yes

Atrial and junctional

PAC and junctional escape

There is a PAC and a junctional escape beat in this tracing. The third P wave is premature and has a different morphology from the two preceding sinus P waves. The next sinus P wave is delayed because of the effects of very marked overdrive suppression. There is a junctional escape beat before this P wave can conduct. The next sinus P wave is also delayed, after which the sinus rhythm increases to about 95 beats/min. Note how the refractory period changes with the heart rate, as reflected in the changing QT intervals.

Tracing 2-36

V$_1$

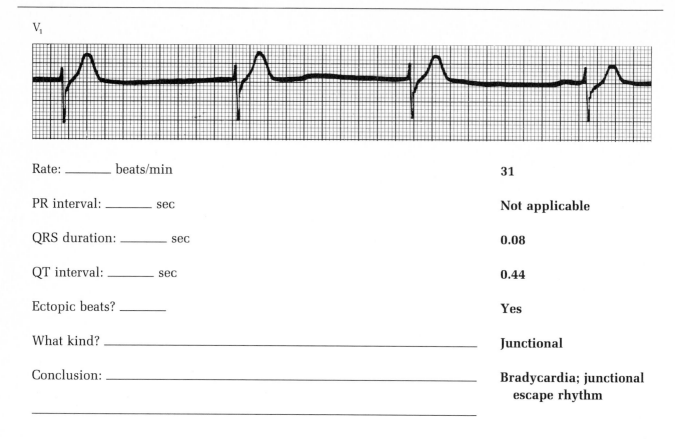

Rate: _____ beats/min

31

PR interval: _____ sec

Not applicable

QRS duration: _____ sec

0.08

QT interval: _____ sec

0.44

Ectopic beats? _____

Yes

What kind? _____

Junctional

Conclusion: _____

Bradycardia; junctional escape rhythm

This is a profound bradycardia and usually requires a pacemaker. In this particular lead there appears to be a junctional escape mechanism. There is no evidence of a P wave; however, you should search all of the other leads before deciding that there indeed are no P waves (atrial stand-still). There may or may not be retrograde activation of the atria during the QRS.

Tracing 2-37

V₁

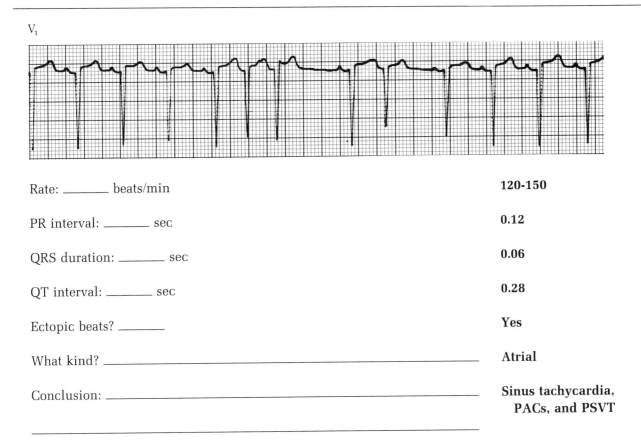

Rate: _____ beats/min   **120-150**

PR interval: _____ sec   **0.12**

QRS duration: _____ sec   **0.06**

QT interval: _____ sec   **0.28**

Ectopic beats? _____   **Yes**

What kind? _____   **Atrial**

Conclusion: _____   **Sinus tachycardia, PACs, and PSVT**

_____

The underlying rhythm here is a sinus tachycardia. There are PACs (sixth and ninth beats), the first of which is followed by a brief, reciprocating mechanism (PSVT).

The combination of myocardial infarction, sinus tachycardia, and frequent PACs should alert you to the possibility of congestive heart failure. The reciprocating mechanism briefly manifested here could be sustained and could produce a ventricular rate in excess of 200 beats/min. This may cause an extension of the infarction. The underlying sinus tachycardia itself contributes to a decrease in cardiac output and coronary perfusion.

Tracing 2-38

II

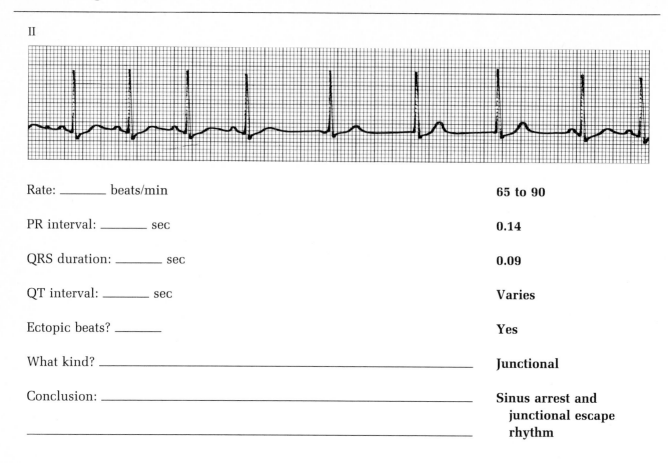

Rate: _____ beats/min   **65 to 90**

PR interval: _____ sec   **0.14**

QRS duration: _____ sec   **0.09**

QT interval: _____ sec   **Varies**

Ectopic beats? _____   **Yes**

What kind? _____   **Junctional**

Conclusion: _____   **Sinus arrest and**
_____   **junctional escape**
                    rhythm

Because of a sudden slowing or arrest of the sinus node there is a junctional escape rhythm for three beats when the sinus node begins firing again. It is, however, only the last P wave that is conducted to the ventricles. The one preceding it is not conducted because the junctional escape beat occurs before it can traverse the AV node and bundle of His. Note that the PR of this beat is shorter than the dominant one and that the ventricular complex is on time with the preceding junctional rhythm.

Tracing 2-39

II

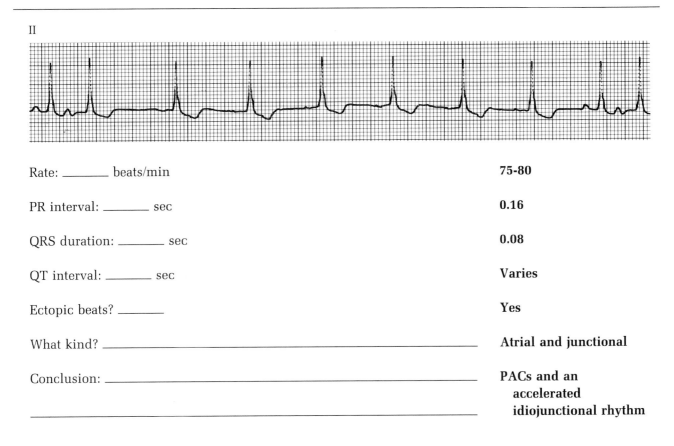

Rate: _____ beats/min — **75-80**

PR interval: _____ sec — **0.16**

QRS duration: _____ sec — **0.08**

QT interval: _____ sec — **Varies**

Ectopic beats? _____ — **Yes**

What kind? _____ — **Atrial and junctional**

Conclusion: _____
_____ — **PACs and an accelerated idiojunctional rhythm**

In this tracing sinus P waves coupled with very early PACs are seen at the beginning and end of the strip. Evidently the PAC suppresses the sinus node enough to unmask an accelerated junctional focus. At first glance the rhythm after the first PAC looks like an escape mechanism. However, a rate of 75 beats/min is too fast for a passive escape response. This arrhythmia may be the result of digitalis toxicity.

3

VENTRICULAR ECTOPICS

☐ **Premature ventricular complexes**

☐ **Ventricular tachycardia**

☐ **Torsades de pointes**

☐ **Ventricular fibrillation**

☐ **Ventricular flutter**

☐ **Accelerated idioventricular rhythm**

☐ **Ventricular escape**

Premature ventricular complexes

Premature ventricular complexes (PVCs) originate in an ectopic focus in the ventricles and are life threatening in the setting of myocardial infarction. They may be the result of a microreentry circuit, automaticity, or afterdepolarizations.

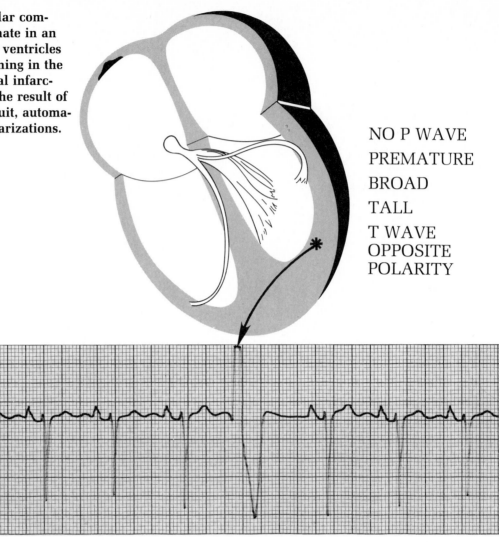

NO P WAVE

PREMATURE

BROAD

TALL

T WAVE OPPOSITE POLARITY

A PVC is recognized because it has _____ _____ _____ wave; it is _____, _____, and _____; and the _____ wave is opposite in polarity to the ventricular complex.

no related P

premature; broad; tall; T

PVCs are life threatening in the setting of _____ _____.

myocardial infarction

R on T

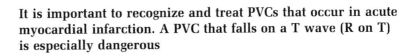

It is important to recognize and treat PVCs that occur in acute myocardial infarction. A PVC that falls on a T wave (R on T) is especially dangerous

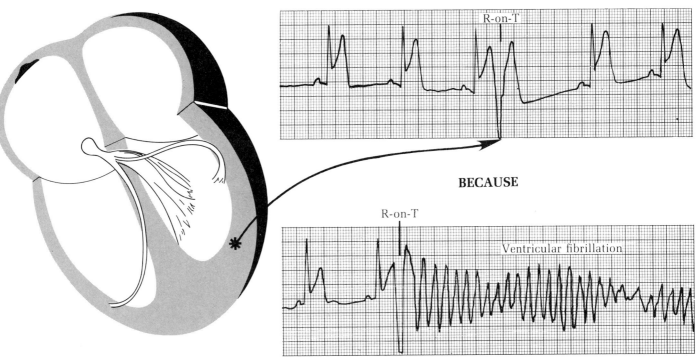

BECOUSE

it may result in ventricular fibrillation or ventricular tachycardia.

"R on T" is a PVC that falls on the _____ _____.

PVCs in myocardial infarction may result in ventricular _____ or _____.

T wave

tachycardia
fibrillation

The full compensatory pause

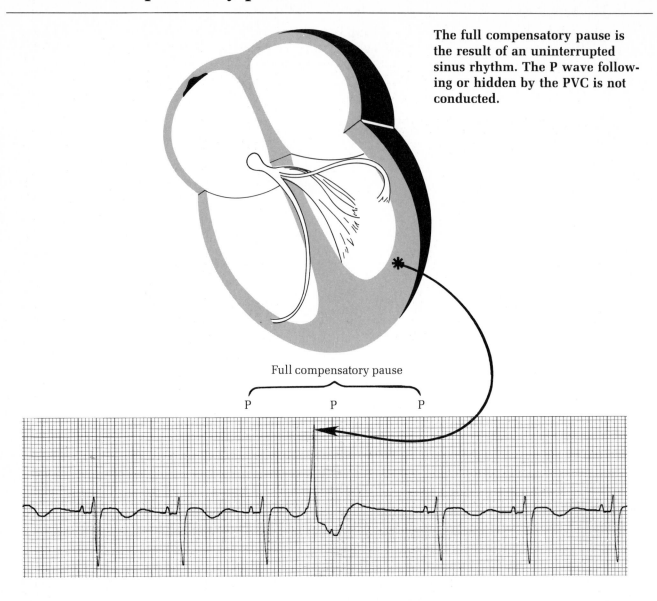

The full compensatory pause is the result of an uninterrupted sinus rhythm. The P wave following or hidden by the PVC is not conducted.

Full compensatory pause

P   P   P

The full compensatory pause supports a diagnosis of ventricular ectopy *only* if the nonconducted _____ wave can be identified as sinus.   **P**

When there is a full compensatory pause, one can "walk out" the _____ waves in spite of the PVC.   **P**

PAC with overdrive suppression

II

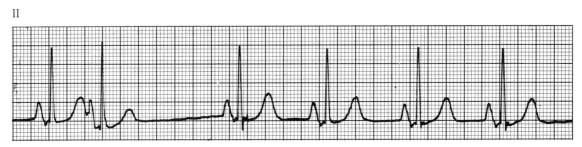

A PAC may cause the next sinus beat to be delayed (overdrive suppression), simulating a full compensatory pause. The sinus beat following the PAC may even be delayed longer (more than full compensatory pause).

II

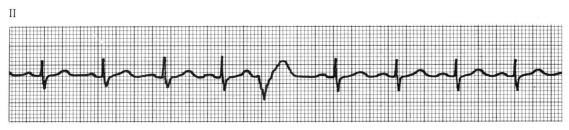

When a PAC is aberrantly conducted *and* has overdrive suppression, it may exactly simulate the PVC with a full compensatory pause.

A full compensatory pause may be seen following _____ and _____.   **PVCs; PACs**

If there is _____ ventricular conduction, a supraventricular complex may be mistaken for a PVC if the full compensatory pause is your only guide.   **aberrant**

NOTE: *A full compensatory pause may also follow a premature junctional beat when retrograde conduction does not occur.*

Ventricular tachycardia

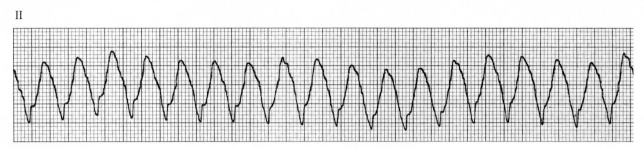

In ventricular tachycardia there is an ectopic focus in the ventricle as a result of automaticity, reentry, or afterdepolarizations. This is a life-threatening arrhythmia.

Ventricular tachycardia is initiated by a _____.   **PVC**

The rate of the ventricular tachycardia above is _____ beats/min.   **165**

This ventricular rhythm is usually _____.   **regular**

Torsades de pointes

II

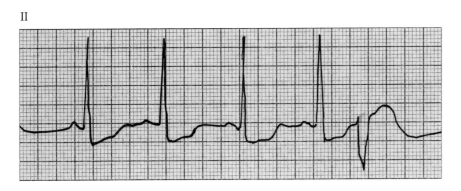

Torsades de pointes (twists of points) is a type of ventricular tachycardia that is often paroxysmal and that occurs in the setting of a long QT interval, which is commonly secondary to therapy with quinidine or quinidine-like drugs (procainamide and disopyramide) but which may also be the result of hypokalemia and complete heart block. The above tracing is from a patient who had been receiving procainamide (500 mg four times a day, orally).

Continuous tracing.

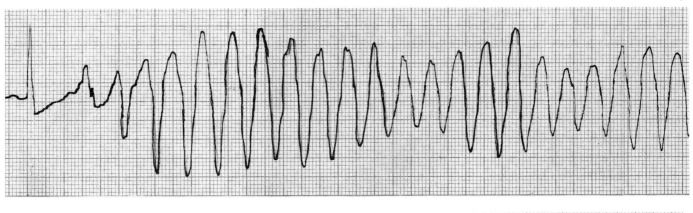

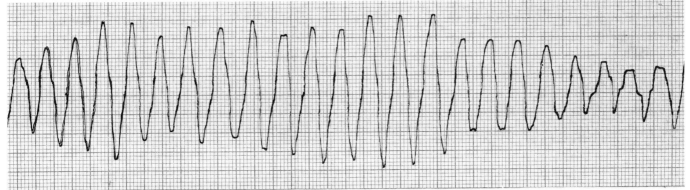

Torsades de pointes (tor-sad d-pwant) is often _____, but may also be sustained. — **paroxysmal**

Torsades de pointes is secondary to _____ QT intervals. — **long**

Torsades de pointes is a type of _____ _____. — **ventricular tachycardia**

The drugs responsible for this arrhythmia are _____, _____, and _____. — **quinidine** **procainamide;** **disopyramide**

Ventricular fibrillation

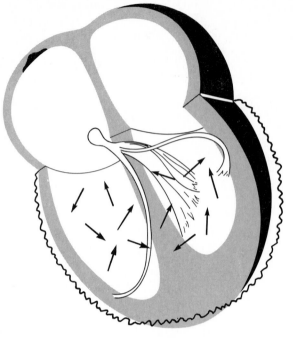

Ventricular fibrillation results when there is electrical chaos in the ventricles. It is initiated by a single PVC or is a deterioration of ventricular tachycardia.

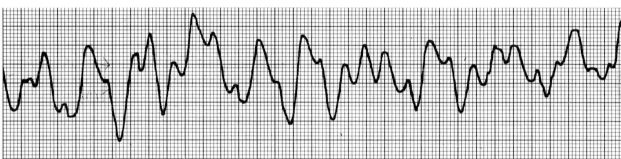

Coarse ventricular fibrillation

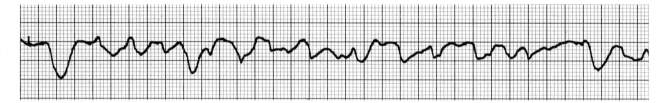

Fine ventricular fibrillation

In ventricular fibrillation the ventricles do not _____.   **pump**

Ventricular fibrillation may be initiated by a single _____.   **PVC**

Ventricular fibrillation may be either coarse or _____.   **fine**

Ventricular fibrillation is easily recognized because it is totally

_____.   **erratic**

Tracing 3-1

II

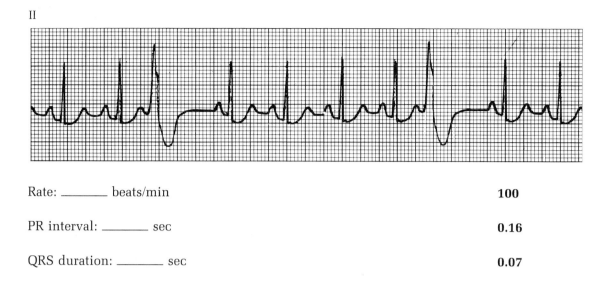

Rate: _____ beats/min   **100**

PR interval: _____ sec   **0.16**

QRS duration: _____ sec   **0.07**

QT interval: _____ sec   **0.32**

Ectopic beats? _____   **Yes**

What kind? _____   **Ventricular**

Conclusion: _____   **PVCs**

You probably had no difficulty in recognizing the two premature ventricular ectopic beats in this tracing. They have all the classic signs of the PVC. There is no related P wave, and they are broad and distorted, with an increased amplitude and a T wave of opposite polarity. Perhaps you also noticed that each PVC is exactly coupled, or linked, to the preceding complex. The coupling interval between the PVC and the preceding complex is 0.36 sec. The interval is exactly the same in both instances, as if the PVC were somehow dependent on the preceding beat for its own generation. It is thought that exact coupling demonstrates a ventricular reentry mechanism or an afterdepolarization. In reentry the sinus-conducted impulse would take the same time each beat to travel through the area of decreased conduction velocity and emerge to recapture the ventricles. If an afterdepolarization were involved, it would be precisely in the same location following the action potential, given a regular underlying rhythm.

Tracing 3-2

II

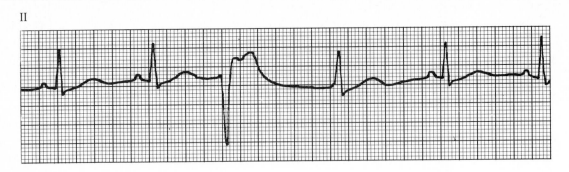

Rate: _____ beats/min   **55 (underlying)**

PR interval: _____ sec   **0.15**

QRS duration: _____ sec   **0.12**

QT interval: _____ sec   **0.52**

Ectopic beats? _____   **Yes**

What kind? _____   **Ventricular and
                                                              junctional**

Conclusion: _____   **Sinus bradycardia;
                                                              junctional escape;
_____   PVC**

Because the underlying rhythm is slow, the compensatory pause after the PVC allows for a junctional escape beat. In this complex the sinus P wave can be seen causing an initial slur in the QRS and making it look broader than it actually is.

The concern here is, of course, the ventricular ectopic beat and not the junctional escape beat. The treatment of this arrhythmia would depend on the clinical picture and how many PVCs were occurring each minute. The bradycardia would not be treated unless the blood pressure were low.

The long QT interval is also cause for alarm, especially if the patient is taking quinidine, procainamide, or disopyramide. Even when the long QT results from bradycardia, torsades de pointes has been reported. A miodarone has also been reported to produce long QT intervals and to cause torsades de pointes.

Tracing 3-3

MCL₁

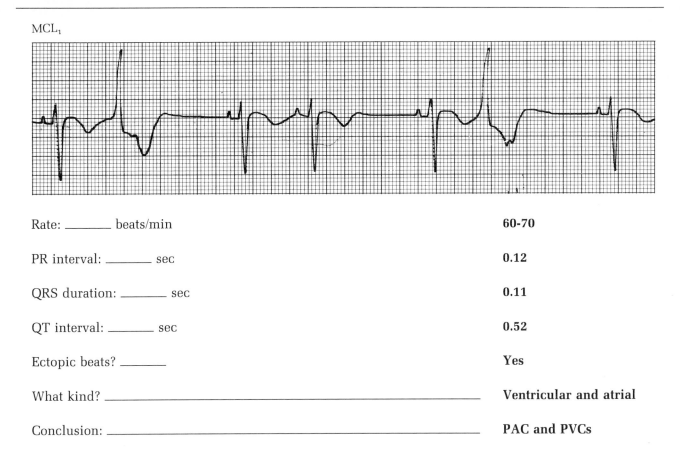

Rate: _____ beats/min   **60-70**

PR interval: _____ sec   **0.12**

QRS duration: _____ sec   **0.11**

QT interval: _____ sec   **0.52**

Ectopic beats? _____   **Yes**

What kind? _____   **Ventricular and atrial**

Conclusion: _____   **PAC and PVCs**

There are atrial and ventricular ectopies in this tracing. The PVCs are the second and sixth beats. The normal sinus P waves can be seen right on time in the T waves of the PVCs. The fourth beat is a PAC. The QT is too long—a warning sign.

Tracing 3-4

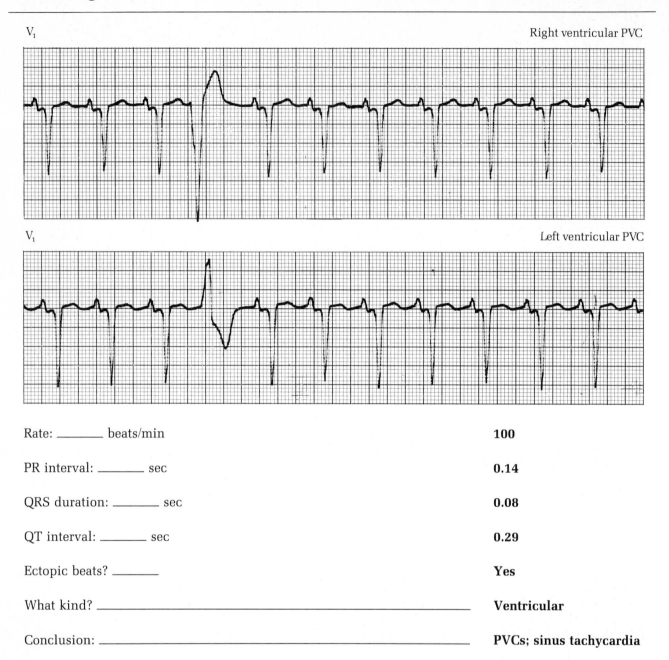

V₁   Right ventricular PVC

V₁   Left ventricular PVC

Rate: _____ beats/min	**100**
PR interval: _____ sec	**0.14**
QRS duration: _____ sec	**0.08**
QT interval: _____ sec	**0.29**
Ectopic beats? _____	**Yes**
What kind? _____	**Ventricular**
Conclusion: _____	**PVCs; sinus tachycardia**

This patient has both right- and left-ventricular PVCs. It is felt that the left-ventricular PVC is more threatening than a PVC from the right ventricle because its location places it closer to the preceding refractory period. However, in the setting of acute myocardial infarction any PVC threatens.

The site of the ventricular ectopic focus is determined by observing the polarity of the ectopic complex in V_1. If the ectopic current originates in the right ventricle, it will proceed to the left and posteriorly, away from the positive electrode of V_1. A negative complex will then be inscribed. Conversely, if the ectopic current originates in the left ventricle, it will proceed toward the positive electrode of V_1. A positive complex will be inscribed.

It is also important to understand what a compensatory pause is and how to use it as a diagnostic aid. In these tracings, the P wave following each PVC is on time. The two PVCs do not interfere with the normal sinus rhythm. There is a pause because the P wave after the PVC (in this case the P wave is buried in the ectopic T wave) is not conducted, as a result of physiological refractoriness. However, to be sure that this is a nonconducted sinus P wave, one must either be able to see it and walk it out or be able to exclude the existence of an ectopic P wave in front of the broad QRS. Remember that a PAC may suppress the sinus node, delaying the next P wave instead of causing it to come earlier as expected. Thus, a PAC can exactly simulate the uninterrupted sinus rhythm that accompanies a PVC. It is apparent then that the presence of a full compensatory pause can mean *either* atrial *or* ventricular ectopy. What then is the value of measuring it at all? When the compensatory pause following an ectopic-looking beat is *less than full*, it is obvious that atrial ectopy is involved and that the sinus node has been "reset." Also, somtimes the sinus P wave immediately following the broad QRS can be identified, proving ventricular ectopy.

Tracing 3-5

II

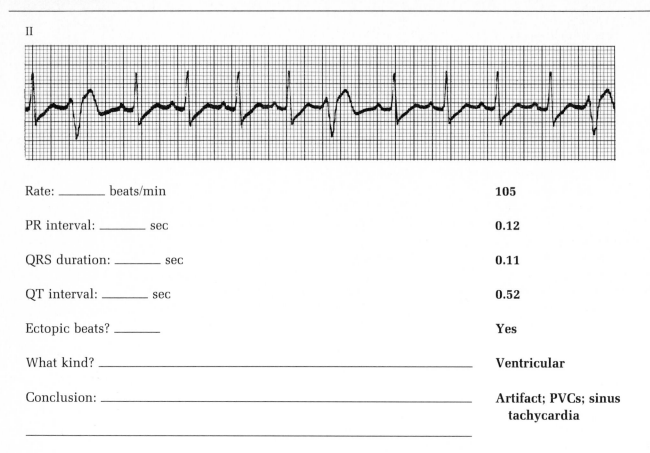

Rate: _____ beats/min   **105**

PR interval: _____ sec   **0.12**

QRS duration: _____ sec   **0.11**

QT interval: _____ sec   **0.52**

Ectopic beats? _____   **Yes**

What kind? _____   **Ventricular**

Conclusion: _____   **Artifact; PVCs; sinus**
                                                                 tachycardia

_____

   In spite of an underlying AC interference throughout the tracing, three
unifocal PVCs are easily seen. The accompanying sinus tachycardia may be
attributed to any of a number of causes (such as fever, emotions, or physical activity). It may also be the response of the sinus node to a failing left
ventricle. A thorough physical assessment should be carried out along with
aggressive treatment of the ventricular ectopics.

Tracing 3-6

V₁

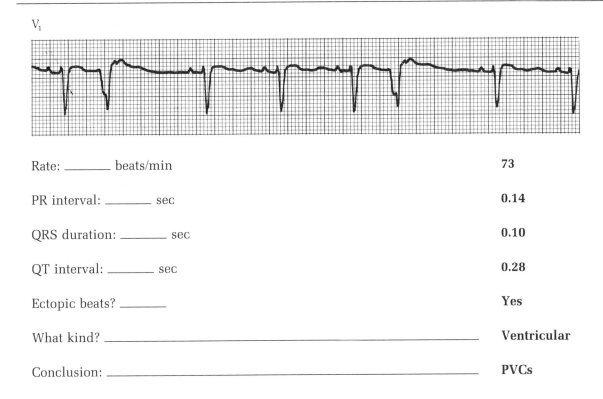

Rate: _____ beats/min

PR interval: _____ sec

QRS duration: _____ sec

QT interval: _____ sec

Ectopic beats? _____

What kind? _____

Conclusion: _____

73

0.14

0.10

0.28

Yes

Ventricular

PVCs

The two PVCs in this tracing have retrograde conduction to the atria. This means that the ventricular ectopic current traveled backward up the AV junction to prematurely invade the atria. This will affect the sinus node jusy as any atrial ectopic stimulus would. Either the sinus node will reset itself, causing the next expected sinus P wave to be earlier, or the P′ wave will cause overdrive suppression, causing a delay in the next sinus discharge.

When you walk out the P waves, you will see that there is less than a full compensatory pause, and yet these are decidedly PVCs. Therefore, when the sinus P wave after an anomalous-looking beat is found to be early (less than full compensatory pause), you are obliged to search not only the T wave preceding the beat in question (to look for a PAC), but also the T wave following such a complex (to look for a retrograde P′).

Tracing 3-7

II

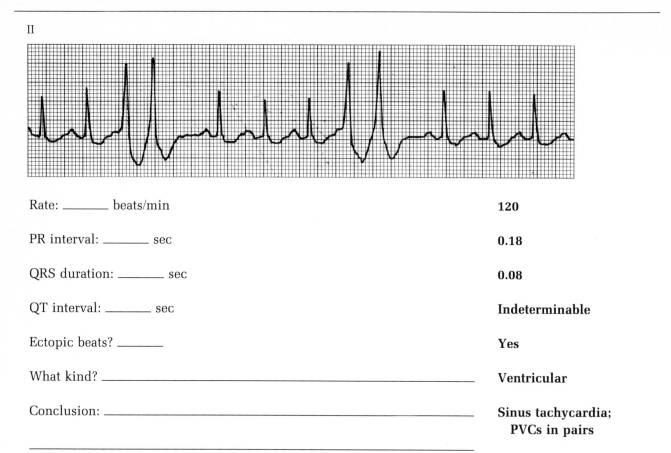

Rate: _____ beats/min

120

PR interval: _____ sec

0.18

QRS duration: _____ sec

0.08

QT interval: _____ sec

Indeterminable

Ectopic beats? _____

Yes

What kind? _____

Ventricular

Conclusion: _____

**Sinus tachycardia;
PVCs in pairs**

The underlying rhythm is a sinus tachycardia, with somatic tremor slightly distorting the ST segments and P waves. There are frequent PVCs (occuring in pairs or "back to back"), which certainly deserve prompt, aggressive treatment. When PVCs follow one another at a rapid rate, each succeeding ectopic beat depolarizes at a lower resting membrane potential, which causes dissimilar refractory periods and sets the ventricles up for fibrillation.

Tracing 3-8

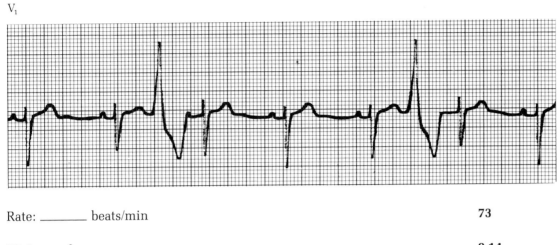

V_1

Rate: _____ beats/min	**73**
PR interval: _____ sec	**0.14**
QRS duration: _____ sec	**0.10**
QT interval: _____ sec	**0.28**
Ectopic beats? _____	**Yes**
What kind? _____	**Ventricular**
Conclusion: _____	**PVCs**

The PVCs in this tracing are called interpolated because they are sandwiched in between two normal sinus-conducted beats without disturbing the rhythm. The interpolated PVC is seen more often in a bradycardia than it is when the underlying rate approaches 70 beats/min., as it does in this tracing.

The changing height of the sinus-conducted ventricular complexes is due to respiration.

The clinical implications of interpolated PVCs are the same as those of any PVC. In the setting of acute myocardial infarction aggressive treatment is indicated.

Tracing 3-9

II

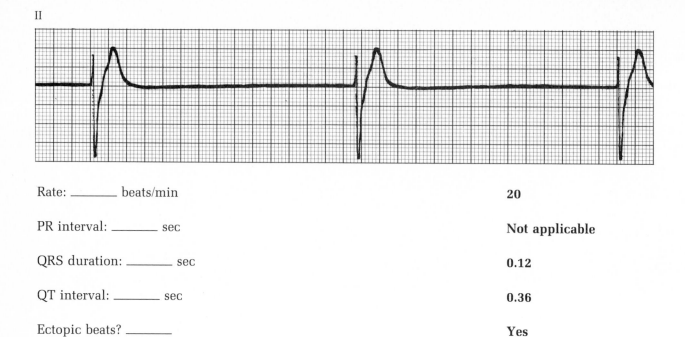

Rate: _____ beats/min   **20**

PR interval: _____ sec   **Not applicable**

QRS duration: _____ sec   **0.12**

QT interval: _____ sec   **0.36**

Ectopic beats? _____   **Yes**

What kind? _____   **Ventricular**

Conclusion: _____   **Slow idioventricular rhythm**

    This tracing represents a very slow idioventricular escape rhythm. No P waves are seen, although another lead might show some. Such a rhythm indicates that all pacemakers above this ventricular focus have failed.

Tracing 3-10

II

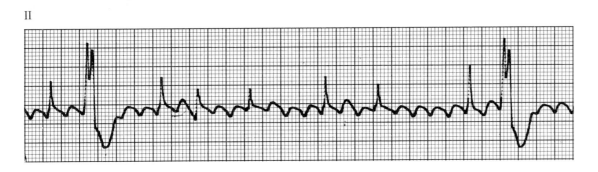

Rate: _____ beats/min

90-100

PR interval: _____ sec

Not applicable

QRS duration: _____ sec

0.08

QT interval: _____ sec

Indeterminable

Ectopic beats? _____

Yes

What kind? _____

Ventricular and atrial

Conclusion: _____

_____

Atrial flutter with variable AV conduction and PVCs

The distinctive sawtooth pattern of atrial flutter is unmistakable in this tracing. There is a variable conduction ratio, sometimes 2:1, 3:1, 4:1, and 5:1. The broad, distorted, ventricular complexes toward the beginning and end of the tracing are probably PVCs.

There is a differential diagnosis between ventricular ectopy and ventricular aberration. The principles governing the morphological distinction between the two are discussed in Chapter 8. (However, they cannot be applied in lead II.)

Tracing 3-11

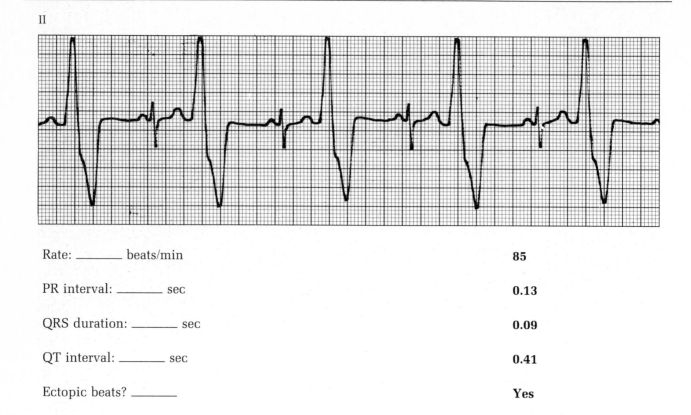

Rate: _____ beats/min   **85**

PR interval: _____ sec   **0.13**

QRS duration: _____ sec   **0.09**

QT interval: _____ sec   **0.41**

Ectopic beats? _____   **Yes**

What kind? _____   **Ventricular**

Conclusion: _____   **Ventricular bigeminy**

When PVCs occur every other beat, as in this tracing, the term "bigeminy" is applied. This tracing gives you an opportunity to note the fixed coupling interval. If you measure the distance between a normally conducted ventricular complex and the PVC that follows it, you will find that the same distance links every couplet in the tracing. This mechanism was explained in the discussion of Tracing 3-1.

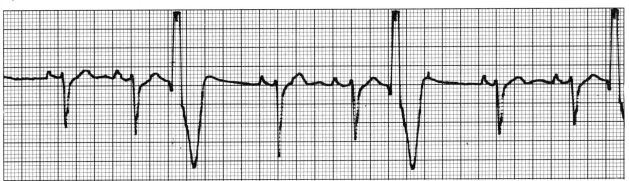

The above figure is an example of trigeminy. There is a PVC every third beat. Both arrhythmias are sometimes seen with digitalis toxicity but may be seen in patients with no symptoms of heart disease.

Tracing 3-12

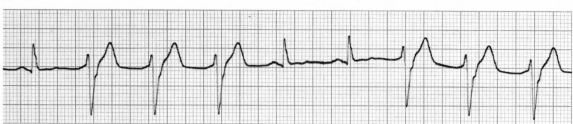

Rate: _____ beats/min	**86-88**
PR interval: _____ sec	**0.14**
QRS duration: _____ sec	**0.09**
QT interval: _____ sec	**0.32**
Ectopic beats? _____	**Yes**
What kind? _____	**Ventricular**
Conclusion: _____	**AIVR**

An accelerated idioventricular rhythm (AIVR) is due to an ectopic focus in the ventricles firing at a enhanced rate (greater than 40 beats/min). Such a focus will usually manifest itself when it achieves the rate of the sinus node and can compete; therefore the AIVR often begins and ends with a fusion beat. Such is not the case in the tracing above. The mechanism of ventricular fusion is discussed and illustrated in Chapter 10, where you will be given practice in recognizing fusion beats.

The AIVR in the tracing below begins with a more premature ventricular ectopic than usual, and yet the rate of the rhythm is slower than the one above, which began with a PVC in the end of the diastolic period.

V_1

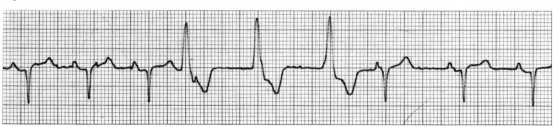

Tracing 3-13

V$_1$

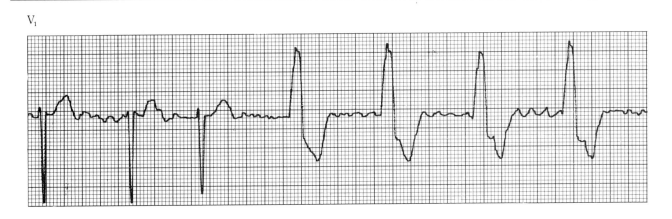

Rate: _____ beats/min   **60-65**

PR interval: _____ sec   **Not applicable**

QRS duration: _____ sec   **0.08**

QT interval: _____ sec   **0.40**

Ectopic beats? _____   **Yes**

What kind? _____   **Ventricular**

Conclusion: _____   **Atrial fibrillation; AIVR**

The underlying rhythm here is atrial fibrillation. There is an accelerated idioventricular focus in the left ventricle that takes over at a rate of 60 beats/min.

At the beginning of the tracing there is an appropriately irregular ventricular response. In atrial fibrillation, absolutely regular and broad ventricular complexes are inappropriate and indicate an idioventricular mechanism. It is "accelerated' because it is faster than the inherent rate of pacemakers below the branching portion of the bundle of His (less than 40 beats/min.)

Tracing 3-14

II   Continuous tracing.

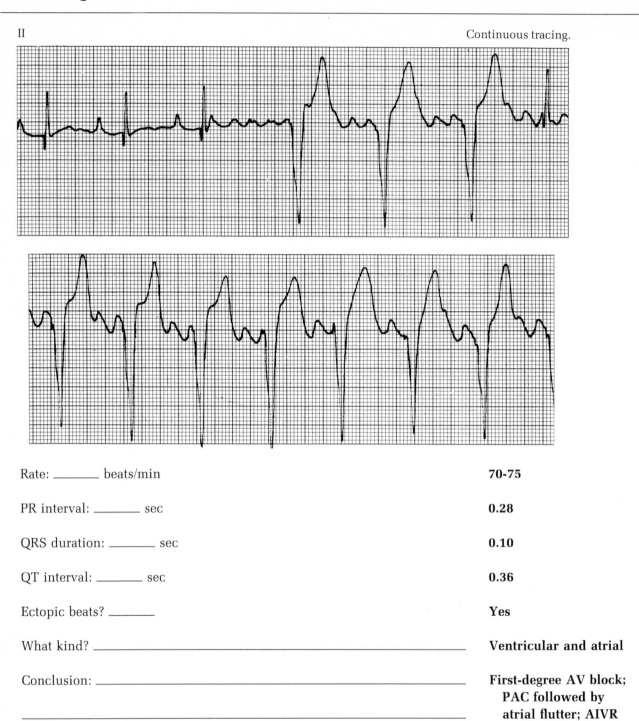

Rate: _____ beats/min   **70-75**

PR interval: _____ sec   **0.28**

QRS duration: _____ sec   **0.10**

QT interval: _____ sec   **0.36**

Ectopic beats? _____   **Yes**

What kind? _____   **Ventricular and atrial**

Conclusion: _____   **First-degree AV block;**
                                                      PAC followed by
_____   **atrial flutter; AIVR**

The accelerated idioventricular rhythm in this tracing occurs against a background of atrial flutter. The beginning of this tracing shows a first degree AV block with normal intraventricular conduction and a prominent U wave, perhaps reflective of hypokalemia. A PAC occurs just after the third ventricular complex and triggers atrial flutter at a rate of 300 beats/min. Killip's rule states that if a premature atrial complex ends a cycle by less than 50%, it is likely to cause a more serious atrial ectopic rhythm. If the P-P' interval is more than 60% of the PP interval, there will be no serious consequences. This rule is certainly well illustrated in this tracing. The P-P' interval is less than 50% of the PP interval, and atrial flutter ensues. The first ventricular complex to occur after the onset of atrial flutter represents an accelerated idioventricular rhythm. One complex can be seen to have been conducted from the atrial pacemaker (capture), but the main ventricular rhythm is dissociated from the atrial rhythm. Even if the onset of the atrial flutter had not been available to you, this diagnosis would still have been evident because of the changing relationship of the flutter wave to the R wave and because of the absolute regularity of the ventricular rhythm. In the bottom half tracing, the flutter waves are not easily seen because of a further acceleration of the ventricular pacemaker. This tracing should impress you with the importance of determining whether the P waves belong to the QRS or not and whether the T waves are all of the same shape. Remember that a P' wave will usually distort a T wave if it occurs at the same time.

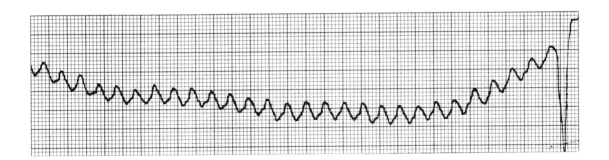

The above tracing is from the same patient after lidocaine was given. Note the disastrous effect of this drug when AV conduction is not normal to begin with (see PR at onset) and when a rapid atrial rate has compounded the AV block. The AIVR was cured, but the patient had no other ventricular rhythm, because of the AV block.

Tracing 3-15

V₁

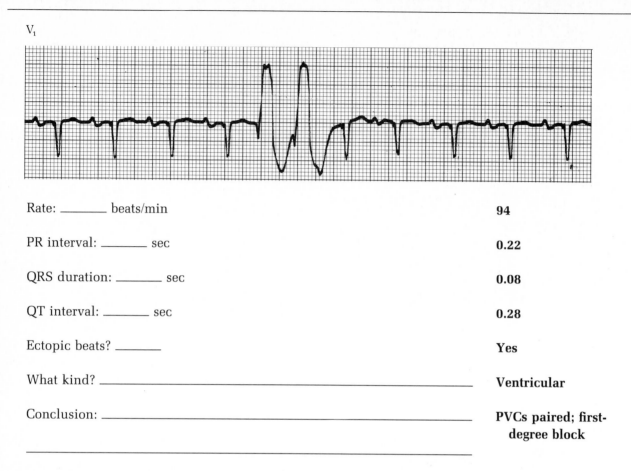

Rate: _____ beats/min   **94**

PR interval: _____ sec   **0.22**

QRS duration: _____ sec   **0.08**

QT interval: _____ sec   **0.28**

Ectopic beats? _____   **Yes**

What kind? _____   **Ventricular**

Conclusion: _____   **PVCs paired; first-
                                                  degree block**
_____

The back-to-back, left-ventricular PVCs in this tracing are a cause for concern and should be treated aggressively. When one PVC follows another in rapid succession, the second of the two is close to the T wave of the preceding beat. This means that it will activate the ventricles when the membrane potential has not yet reached its optimal level for normal uniform conduction. Ventricular fibrillation may be the result of such a sequence, especially in the clinical setting of acute myocardial infarction. The second PVC has retrograde conduction to the atria. The normal complex following it is a reciprocal beat.

This patient also has a first-degree heart block, detected by measuring the PR interval, which should not exceed 0.20 sec. Heart block is discussed and illustrated in Chapter 4.

Tracing 3-16

V₁

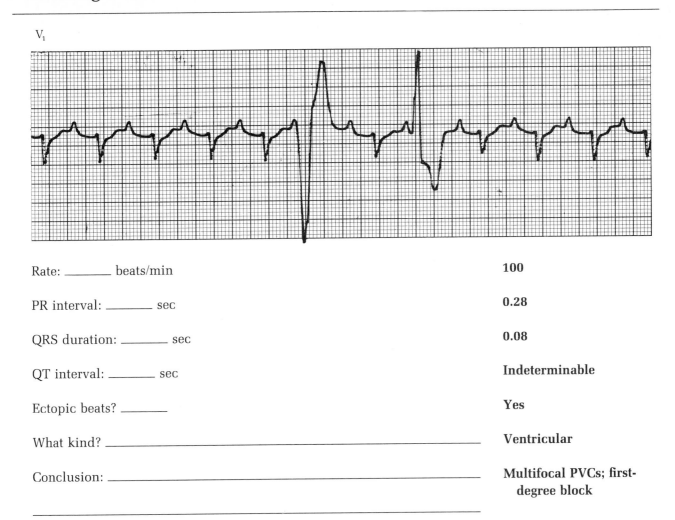

Rate: _____ beats/min   **100**

PR interval: _____ sec   **0.28**

QRS duration: _____ sec   **0.08**

QT interval: _____ sec   **Indeterminable**

Ectopic beats? _____   **Yes**

What kind? _____   **Ventricular**

Conclusion: _____   **Multifocal PVCs; first-
                                                            degree block**

_____

The two PVCs in this tracing are decidedly from different foci. Multifocal PVCs are more threatening than unifocal ones and, in the clinical setting of acute myocardial infarction, should be treated aggressively. The first PVC is right ventricular in origin, and the second is left ventricular. Both of them occur toward the end of diastole. Because this patient also has first-degree heart block with a PR interval of 0.28 sec, there is no chance of the second PVC being a fusion beat. In order for fusion to occur, the ventricular ectopic beat cannot be more than 0.06 or 0.07 sec premature. The second PVC is 0.16 sec premature and completely captures the ventricles before the sinus P wave can conduct across the AV node.

Tracing 3-17

V₁

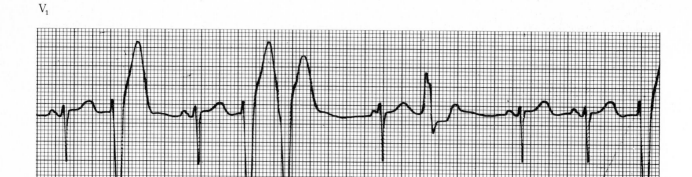

Rate: _____ beats/min

90

PR interval: _____ sec

0.12

QRS duration: _____ sec

0.09

QT interval: _____ sec

0.36

Ectopic beats? _____

Yes

What kind? _____

Ventricular

Conclusion: _____

Multifocal, paired, frequent PVCs

The ventricular ectopy manifested in this tracing is primarily right ventricular; however, because the ectopic beats occur in pairs, are so frequent, and are multifocal (left ventricular as well), treatment will be aggressive.

There is a junctional escape beat following the back-to-back PVCs.

Tracing 3-18

V₁

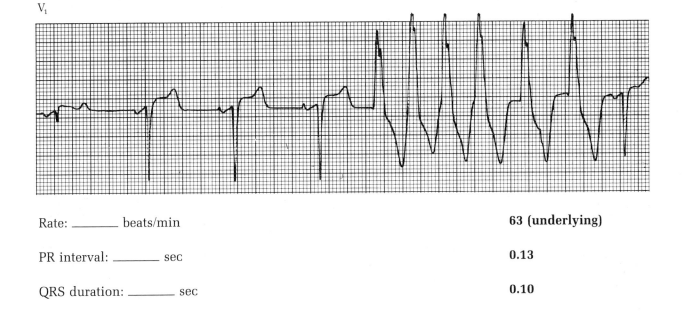

Rate: _____ beats/min   **63 (underlying)**

PR interval: _____ sec   **0.13**

QRS duration: _____ sec   **0.10**

QT interval: _____ sec   **0.40**

Ectopic beats? _____ sec   **Yes**

What kind? _____   **Ventricular**

Conclusion: _____   **Ventricular tachycardia**

This is a paroxysmal left-ventricular tachycardia. The very first complex is a fusion beat. Notice how narrow it is and how decreased the amplitude is compared with the three sinus-conducted beats that follow. A burst of ventricular tachycardia follows. There is a P wave seen immediately after the last ventricular ectopic beat. It probably represents retrograde conduction from the ventricles. It is followed by normal ventricular conduction, in this case a reciprocal beat, which terminates the tachycardia.

Tracing 3-19

II

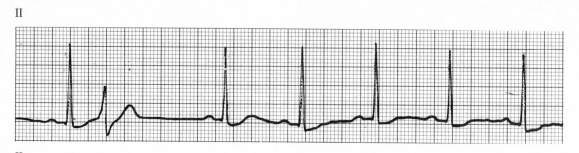

II

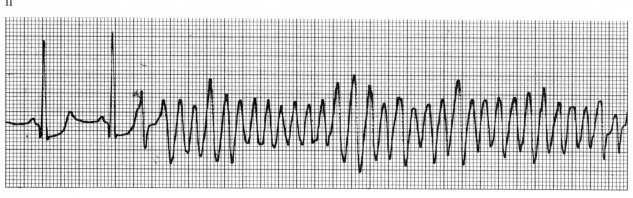

Patient is taking quinidine.

Rate: _____ beats/min   **74 (underlying)**

PR interval: _____ sec   **0.20**

QRS duration: _____ sec   **0.08**

QT interval: _____ sec   **0.56**

Ectopic beats? _____   **Yes**

What kind? _____   **Ventricular**

Conclusion: _____   **Torsades de pointes**

Notice the long QT interval, which is distorted by a U wave. Prior to the tracing seen at the top, this patient had frequent episodes of R-on-T phenomenon. The one that triggered the ventricular tachycardia had the shortest coupling interval of all. Notice the undulating character of the tachycardia.

This arrhythmia does not respond to antiarrhythmic drugs. Additional quinidine or quinidine-like drugs will only compound the matter, and lidocaine and lidocaine-like drugs are unpredictable and may causes harm. It is necessary for the QT to be shortened. This can of course be accomplished by withholding the quinidine. Atrial or ventricular overdrive pacing may be necessary to support the patient until he can metabolize and excrete the offending drug. Successful treatment has also been reported with magnesium sulfate.

Remember that this condition is diagnosed only against a background of long QT intervals. Note the tachycardia on p. 81. It looks like torsades de points, but is not and therefore requires lidocaine.

For further discussion of torsades de pointes, see p. 85.

Tracing 3-20

V$_1$

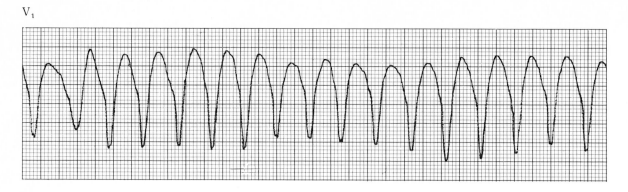

Rate: _____ beats/min

170

PR interval: _____ sec

Not applicable

QRS duration: _____ sec

0.16

QT interval: _____ sec

0.36

Ectopic beats? _____

Yes

What kind? _____

Ventricular

Conclusion: _____

Ventricular tachycardia

Ventricular tachycardia is an extreme emergency. A tachycardia will severely compromise the already ischemic myocardium, depreciate general hemodynamics, and precipitate ventricular fibrillation. The mechanism involved is either (1) a single focus with enhanced automaticity or (2) a reentry mechanism. In the latter case the episode would have been sparked by a single PVC, occurring at just the right time in the cardiac cycle.

Tracing 3-21

V₁

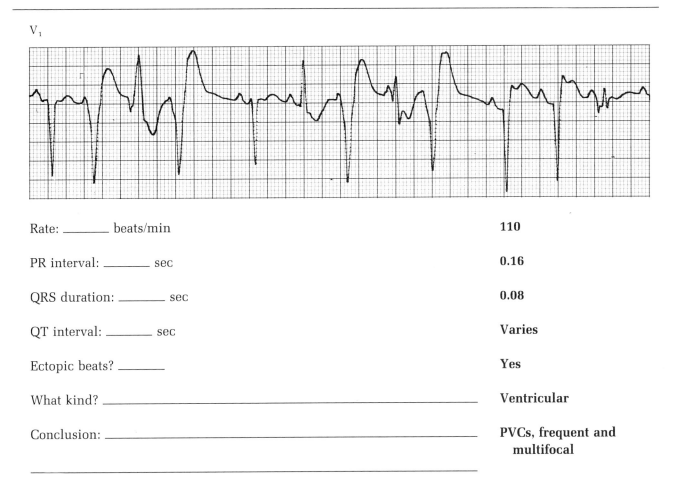

Rate: _____ beats/min   **110**

PR interval: _____ sec   **0.16**

QRS duration: _____ sec   **0.08**

QT interval: _____ sec   **Varies**

Ectopic beats? _____   **Yes**

What kind? _____   **Ventricular**

Conclusion: _____   **PVCs, frequent and multifocal**

There are frequent multifocal PVCs in this tracing. Sometimes they are end-diastolic fusion beats, and therefore it is difficult to pick out the sinus-conducted beats. There is a sinus-conducted beat at the very beginning of the tracing. The fifth beat from the beginning is also a sinus-conducted beat. Evidence of the dual focus is seen right after the first normal beat. There is a right- and then a left-ventricular PVC. Another right-ventricular PVC follows, and it almost looks as though you will see an established bidirectional ventricular tachycardia, which is commonly caused by digitalis toxicity.

Some authorities do not use the term "multifocal" but prefer "multiform" instead. They feel that ventricular ectopics exhibiting more than one morphology in the same heart may actually be one focus with different wave fronts.

4
ATRIOVENTRICULAR BLOCK

- [ ] **First-degree AV block**
- [ ] **Second-degree AV block**
- [ ] **2:1 conduction**
- [ ] **Third-degree AV block**

Sequence of atrioventricular activation

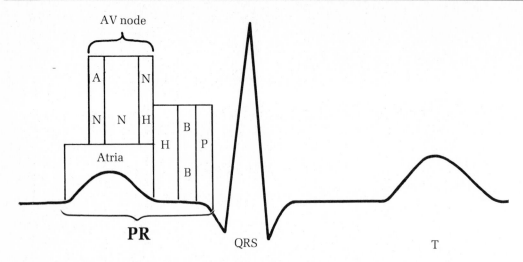

The PR interval reflects conduction time of the cardiac impulse through the atria, AV node, His bundle *(H)*, bundle branches *(BB)*, and Purkinje fibers *(P)*. When the PR interval is long, it is usually the result of conduction delay in the AV node. *AN*, Atrionodal; *N*, node; *NH*, nodal-His.

The AV node is activated about midway through the _____ wave. **P**

The impulse has arrived in the _____ _____ by the time the P wave has been completed. **His bundle**

During the PR segment (from the end of the P to the beginning of the QRS) the _____ _____ are activated. **bundle branches**

First-degree AV block

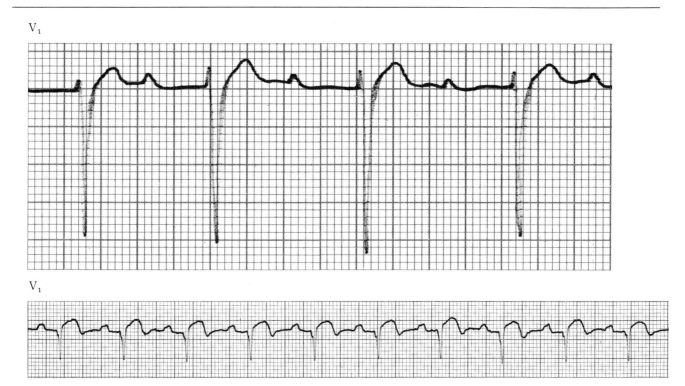

V₁

V₁

In first-degree AV block the PR interval is longer than one large square (0.20 sec).

A PR greater than 0.20 sec constitutes _____-degree AV block.　　**first**

The PR interval in the top tracing is _____ sec.　　**0.36**

The PR interval in the bottom tracing is _____ sec.　　**0.22**

In first-degree AV block the delay is usually in the _____ node.　　**AV**

Type I second-degree AV block (Wenckebach)

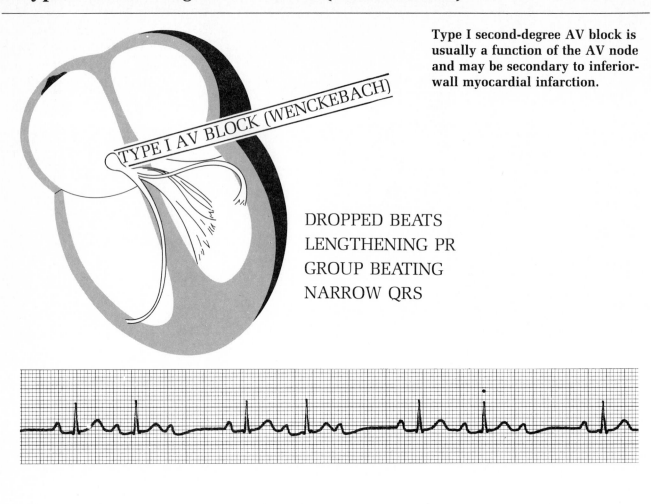

Type I second-degree AV block is usually a function of the AV node and may be secondary to inferior-wall myocardial infarction.

TYPE I AV BLOCK (WENCKEBACH)

DROPPED BEATS
LENGTHENING PR
GROUP BEATING
NARROW QRS

In type I second-degree AV block:

Some sinus P waves are _____ _____.

not conducted

There are lengthening _____ intervals.

PR

There is _____ beating.

group

The QRS is usually _____.

narrow

Type I second-degree AV block is sometimes called _____.

AV Wenckebach

AV Wenckebach is often secondary to _____ _____ myocardial infarction.

inferior-wall

Type II second-degree AV block

In type II second-degree AV block the pathology is in the bundle branches and is usually secondary to anterior septal myocardial infarction.

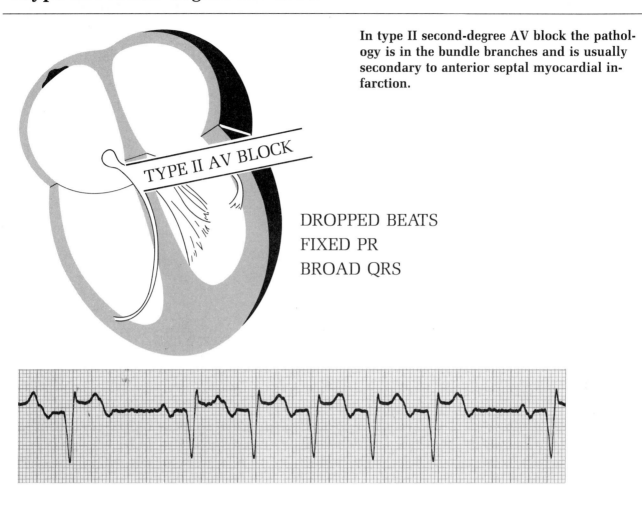

TYPE II AV BLOCK

DROPPED BEATS
FIXED PR
BROAD QRS

In type II second-degree AV block:

Some sinus P waves are _____ _____.   **not conducted**

The _____ intervals are all the same.   **PR**

The QRS is usually _____.   **broad**

2:1 AV conduction

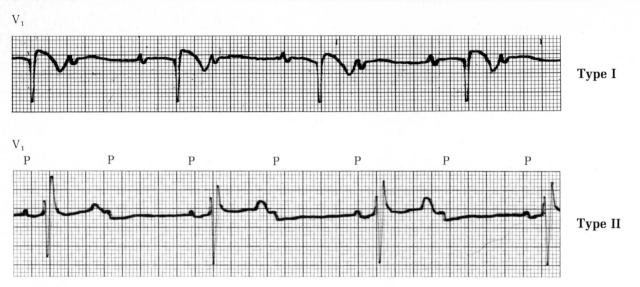

V_1 Type I

V_1 Type II

When the conduction ratio is 2:1, the arrhythmia could be either type I or type II second-degree AV block.

These are your clues:

In type I the QRS is usually _____. **narrow**

In type II the QRS is usually _____. **broad**

Type I will respond to atropine; type II _____ _____. **will not**

Type I is in the setting of _____ -wall myocardial infarction. **inferior**

Type II is in the setting of _____ -wall myocardial infarction. **anterior**

In type I the PR interval is often _____. **long**

In type II the PR interval is often _____. **normal**

Third-degree (complete) AV block

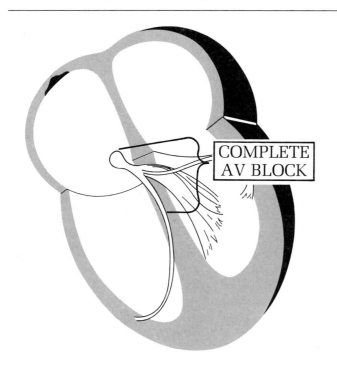

COMPLETE AV BLOCK

Third-degree (complete) AV block may occur at the level of the AV node, the bundle of His, or the bundle branches.

When AV block is complete, there is AV dissociation because of a pathological block in conduction between the _____ and the _____.

atria
ventricles

If the block is in the AV node, the escape pacemaker will be in the _____ _____ _____.

bundle of His

If the block is in the bundle of His, the escape pacemaker will be in the bundle of His below the block or in the _____ _____, depending on the level of the block.

bundle branches

If the escape pacemaker is in the bundle of His, the resulting rhythm is called a _____ escape rhythm; if the escape pacemaker is in the bundle branches, the rhythm is called a _____ escape rhythm.

junctional
ventricular

The QRS will be _____ with a junctional pacemaker and _____ with a ventricular pacemaker.

narrow
broad

The rate will be faster and more dependable with a _____ pacemaker; it will be slower and less dependable with a _____ pacemaker.

junctional
ventricular

Complete AV block at the level of the bundle branches is called _____ block.

trifascicular

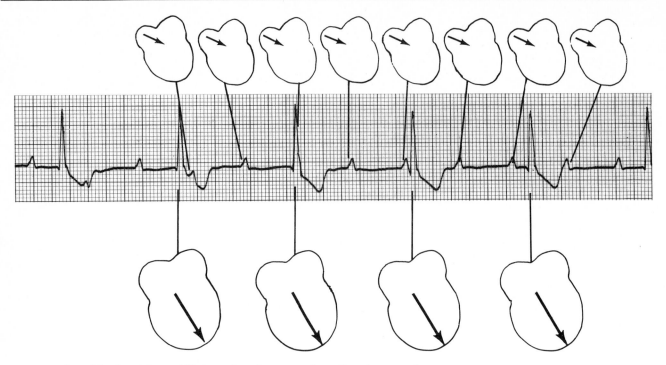

In complete block with an idiojunctional pacemaker the sinus node
paces the atria and the AV junction paces the ventricles.

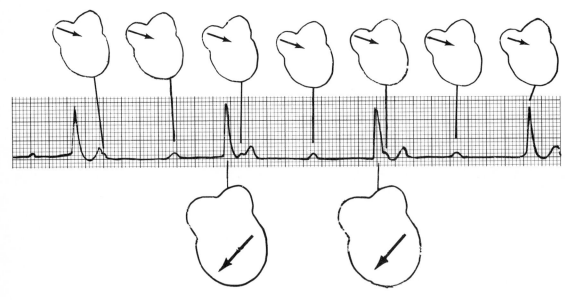

In complete block with an idioventricular pacemaker the sinus node
paces the atria and a ventricular focus paces the ventricles.

Tracing 4-1

V₁

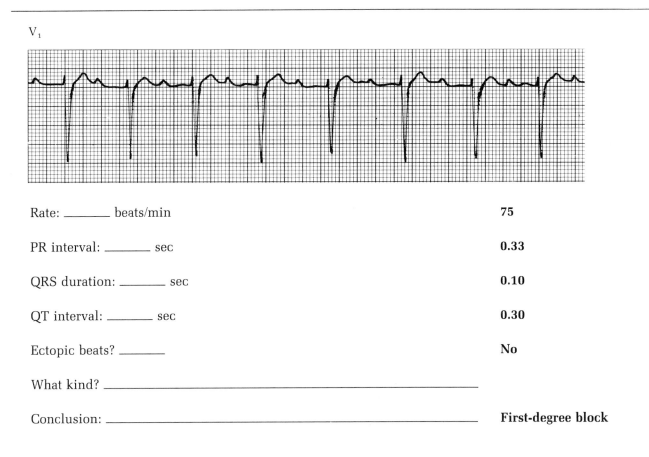

Rate: _____ beats/min   **75**

PR interval: _____ sec   **0.33**

QRS duration: _____ sec   **0.10**

QT interval: _____ sec   **0.30**

Ectopic beats? _____   **No**

What kind? _____

Conclusion: _____   **First-degree block**

Because the PR interval is so long in this tracing, it almost looks as if the P wave belongs to the preceding QRS. However, the slight sinus arrhythmia shows us that the P wave has a constant relationship to the following ventricular complex. This is unmistakably a first-degree heart block.

Tracing 4-2

II

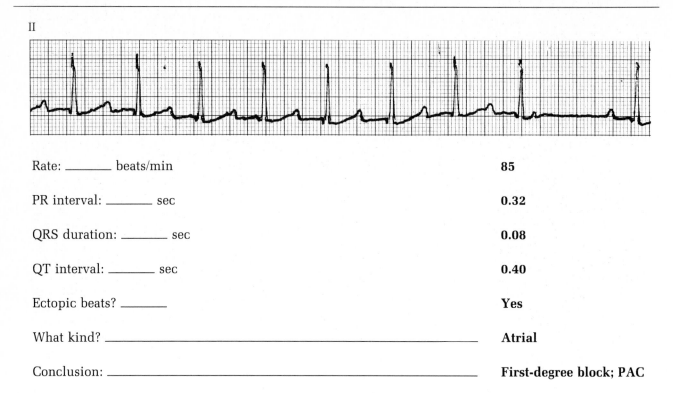

Rate: _____ beats/min	**85**
PR interval: _____ sec	**0.32**
QRS duration: _____ sec	**0.08**
QT interval: _____ sec	**0.40**
Ectopic beats? _____	**Yes**
What kind? _____	**Atrial**
Conclusion: _____	**First-degree block; PAC**

Here is a first-degree heart block with marked lengthening of the PR interval. The rhythm is abruptly interrupted by a nonconducted PAC, which distorts the T wave before the pause. The P wave after the pause may or may not be conducted. It has a shorter PR interval than the others and may therefore represent a junctional escape beat or an improvement in conduction with the longer cycle length.

As you examine this tracing and the preceding one, keep in mind that when a P wave falls midway between two R waves, there is a chance that there is a hidden P' wave and that the rhythm is really an atrial tachycardia with 2:1 block. Carefully examine the QRS-T for any signs of distortion. In this case the nonconducted P' wave seen interrupting the sinus rhythm rules out this possibility.

Tracing 4-3

II

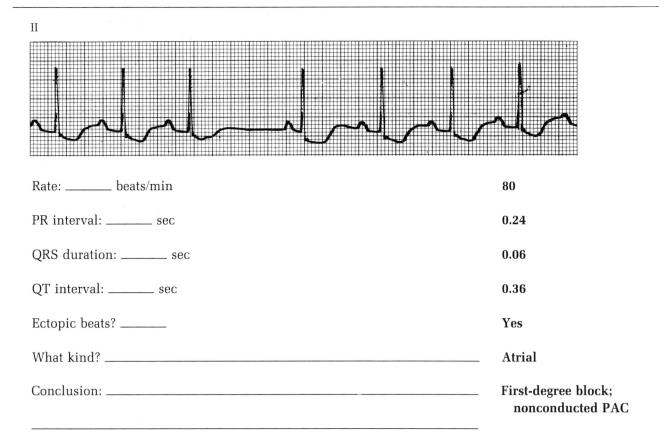

Rate: _____ beats/min   **80**

PR interval: _____ sec   **0.24**

QRS duration: _____ sec   **0.06**

QT interval: _____ sec   **0.36**

Ectopic beats? _____   **Yes**

What kind? _____   **Atrial**

Conclusion: _____   **First-degree block;
                                                     nonconducted PAC**

_____

This tracing represents first-degree heart block with a nonconducted PAC followed by an escape atrial complex. The arrhythmia looks like SA block; however, on close examination, the ST segment just preceding the pause is found to have a little bump in it. When you compare this ST segment with the two preceding ones, you will easily see the P' wave, which is not conducted because it is so premature that the AV junction is still refractory.

Here, as in Tracing 4-2, the PR interval following the pause is shorter than all of the others, and the same possibilities exist: a junctional escape beat fires before the P wave can conduct or the first-degree AV block is relieved by the longer cycle length.

Tracing 4-4

V$_1$

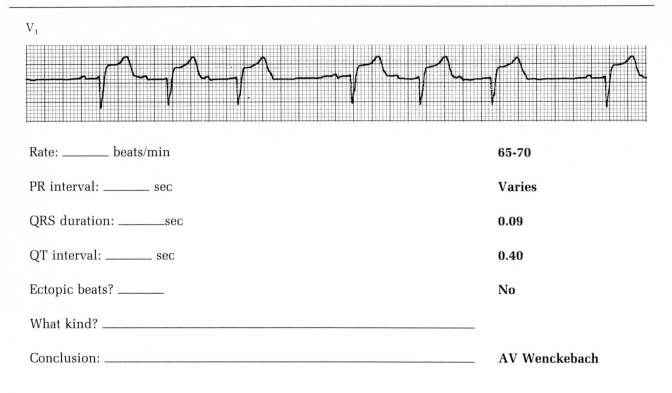

Rate: _____ beats/min

65-70

PR interval: _____ sec

Varies

QRS duration: _____ sec

0.09

QT interval: _____ sec

0.40

Ectopic beats? _____

No

What kind? _____

Conclusion: _____

AV Wenckebach

Here again is the group beating that is so characteristic of Wenckebach. In this case of type I second-degree heart block the conduction ratio is 4:3; that is, for every four P waves, three of them are conducted. If you start at the beginning of the tracing and walk out the P waves, you will find the fourth P wave of each set (right on time) distorting the third T wave of that set.

Tracing 4-5

III

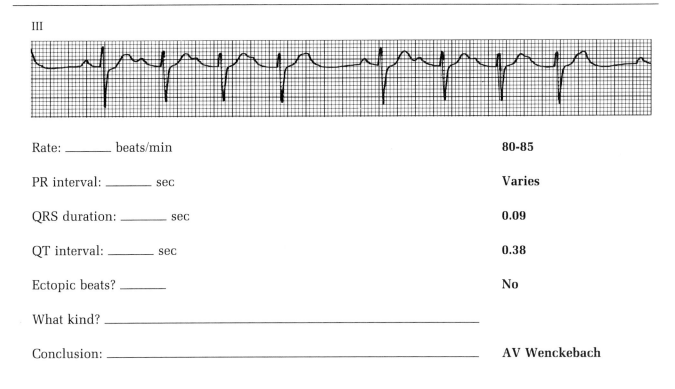

Rate: _____ beats/min — **80-85**

PR interval: _____ sec — **Varies**

QRS duration: _____ sec — **0.09**

QT interval: _____ sec — **0.38**

Ectopic beats? _____ — **No**

What kind? _____

Conclusion: _____ — **AV Wenckebach**

This is AV Wenckebach 5:4. The P waves are not as easily seen in this tracing. However, group beating will alert you to the possibility of Wenckebach conduction. The first two P waves are noticeable. If you walk them out, you will find all of the others on time and distorting T waves.

When the diagnosis of an arrhythmia is not immediately self-evident, maintain a standard approach. First, what is the sinus node doing? Second, establish whether or not there is AV conduction. An irregular rhythm indicates some conduction, since an idioventricular or idiojunctional rhythm would be absolutely regular. Finally, measure the PR intervals. In this case you cannot help but come up with the diagnosis of lengthening PR intervals and dropped beats (Wenckebach).

There is another sign of Wenckebach in this tracing—shortening RR intervals.

Tracing 4-6

II

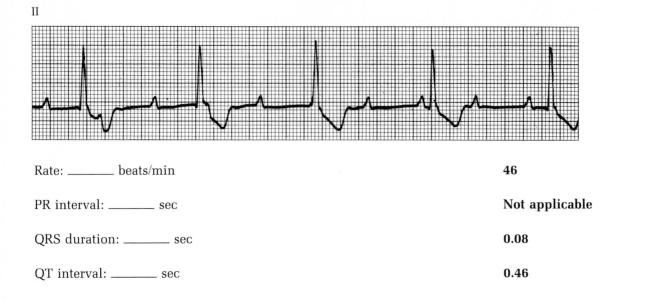

Rate: _____ beats/min   **46**

PR interval: _____ sec   **Not applicable**

QRS duration: _____ sec   **0.08**

QT interval: _____ sec   **0.46**

Ectopic beats? _____   **Yes**

What kind? _____   **Junctional**

Conclusion: _____   **Complete AV block**

Did you fall into the trap of calling this a second-degree heart block with 2:1 AV conduction? Whenever you make such a diagnosis, follow it up by making sure that all of the PR intervals are the same. In this case they are not. This is a complete, or third-degree, heart block with an idiojunctional rhythm. The ventricular rate is 46 beats/min, and the atrial rate is 100. An idiojunctional rhythm is distinguished from an idioventricular rhythm by the duration of the QRS complex. If the ventricles are paced by the AV junction, the QRS will be normal. If the pacemaker is below the branching portion of the bundle of His, the QRS will be broad and the rate will be slower and less dependable then that of an idiojunctional pacemaker. In this arrhythmia the atria and the ventricles beat entirely independently of each other, which means that some of the R waves may be superimposed on a P wave. In this tracing all the P waves except one are visible. There is one distorting the first and second ST segments and one hidden by the third R wave.

Tracing 4-7

II

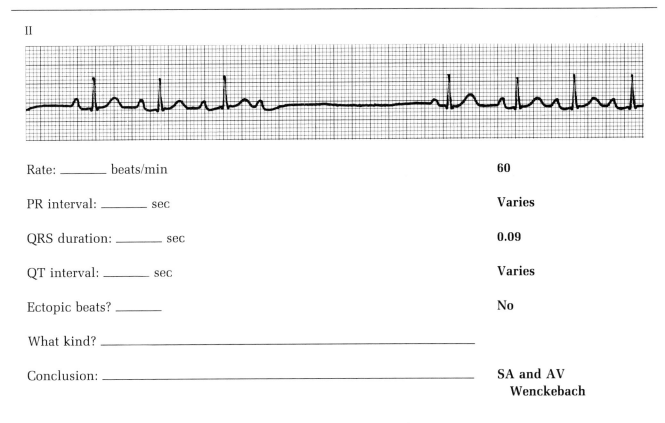

Rate: _____ beats/min   **60**

PR interval: _____ sec   **Varies**

QRS duration: _____ sec   **0.09**

QT interval: _____ sec   **Varies**

Ectopic beats? _____   **No**

What kind? _____

Conclusion: _____ **SA and AV**
                                              Wenckebach

This is a type I (Wenckebach) second-degree AV block with SA block. However, there is an additional problem. You will notice that the PP intervals are shortening before the long pause. This indicates a Wenckebach of the sinus node as well. The shortening occurs because the largest increment in conduction from the sinus node to the atrial tissue is between the first and second P waves of the group. The typical Wenckebach, whether it is from the sinus node or the AV node, will have shortening RR intervals. It should be noted, however, that not all Wenckebachs are typical.

Tracing 4-8

V$_1$

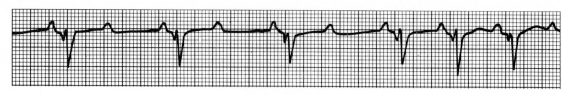

Rate: _____ beats/min   **60**

PR interval: _____ sec   **0.14**

QRS duration: _____ sec   **0.14**

QT interval: _____ sec   **Indeterminable**

Ectopic beats? _____   **No**

What kind? _____

Conclusion: _____   **Type II second-degree
                                                     AV block**

_____

This is a type II second-degree AV block. The last part of the tracing gives an opportunity to see two or more conducted beats in a row and thus rule out AV Wenckebach. Type II AV block is usually accompanied by a broad QRS complex, since the lesion is below the branching portion of the bundle of His. Type II AV block is associated with a less favorable prognosis than is the Wenckebach type and almost always requires a pacemaker.

Tracing 4-9

II

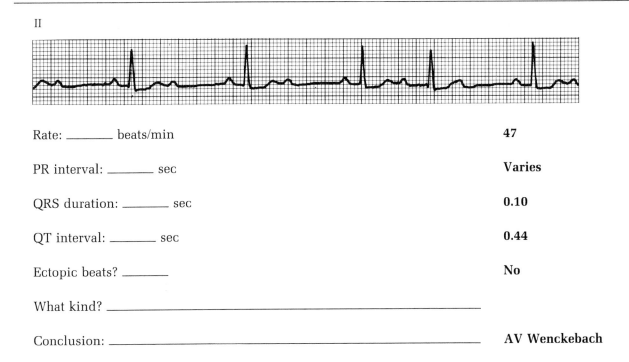

Rate: _____ beats/min   **47**

PR interval: _____ sec   **Varies**

QRS duration: _____ sec   **0.10**

QT interval: _____ sec   **0.44**

Ectopic beats? _____   **No**

What kind? _____

Conclusion: _____   **AV Wenckebach**

This is second-degree AV block, type I. The beginning of this tracing shows 2:1 AV conduction (that is, two P waves for every QRS complex) and a PR interval of 0.20 sec. However, if you look at the group of complexes at the end of the strip, you will see that there is a PR interval of 0.20 sec, followed by another conducted P wave with a PR interval of 0.30 sec, and then a P wave (on the T) that is not conducted. This lengthening of the PR interval with a nonconducted beat constitutes type I (Wenckebach) second-degree AV block. When there are three P waves for two ventricular complexes, a 3:2 conduction is said to exist. As long as there are two conducted P waves in a row, you will have no difficulty in diagnosing the type of block. However, when there is 2:1 conduction (every other P wave), one relies on other clues to help in the differential diagnosis. The duration of the QRS complex can be of some help to you in this dilemma. It has been shown that type I is a function of the AV node. The lengthening PR intervals would then be accompanied by a narrow QRS complex. Type II almost always involves a lesion lower in the conductive system, at the branching portion of the bundle of His, and hence is accompanied by a broad QRS complex. In this tracing, if you did not have the two conducted P waves in a row to go by, the narrow QRS would favor type I, as would the normal PR interval.

Tracing 4-10

V$_1$

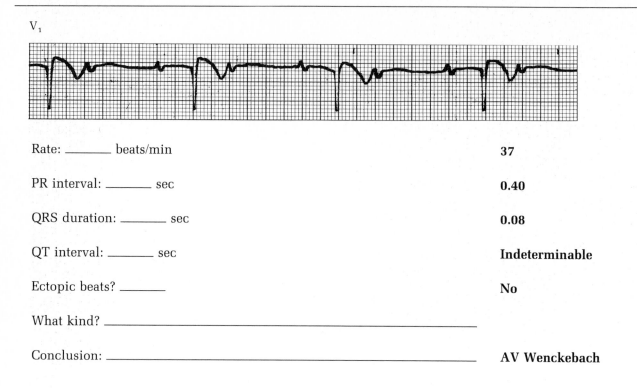

Rate: _____ beats/min

PR interval: _____ sec

QRS duration: _____ sec

QT interval: _____ sec

Ectopic beats? _____

What kind? _____

Conclusion: _____

37

0.40

0.08

Indeterminable

No

AV Wenckebach

This is a second-degree AV block, type I, with 2:1 AV conduction. Since there are not two conducted beats in a row, we are unable to determine whether the PR interval is lengthening. However, since the QRS duration is normal, we know that the block is above the branching portion of the bundle of His and we can therefore assume that the block is of the AV node. Note also the long PR interval, another sign of type I AV block.

Tracing 4-11

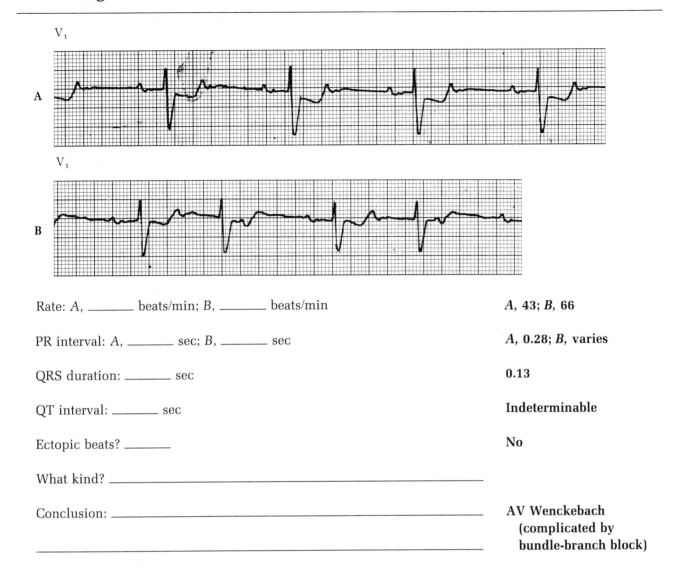

Rate: A, _____ beats/min; B, _____ beats/min   **A, 43; B, 66**

PR interval: A, _____ sec; B, _____ sec   **A, 0.28; B, varies**

QRS duration: _____ sec   **0.13**

QT interval: _____ sec   **Indeterminable**

Ectopic beats? _____   **No**

What kind? _____

Conclusion: _____   **AV Wenckebach (complicated by bundle-branch block)**

_____

This is a type I second-degree AV block complicated by bundle-branch block. In the second tracing, which is from the same patient as the first, two consecutive conducted beats are seen, with PR intervals lengthening from 0.32 to 0.44 sec. The third P wave is then not conducted, constituting a Wenckebach phenomenon. If only the first tracing were available, you would be quite justified in presuming this to be a type II AV block, since the QRS duration is prolonged. This lengthening, in addition to the long PR interval, would cause you to anticipate more serious conduction disturbances, since the lesion probably involves more than one area of the conductive system—the AV node and the bundle branches.

Tracing 4-12

II

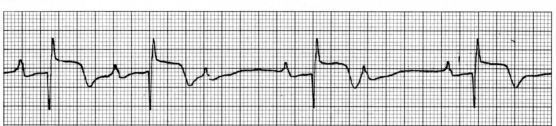

Rate: _____ beats/min   **45**

PR interval: _____ sec   **Varies**

QRS duration: _____ sec   **0.10**

QT interval: _____ sec   **0.58**

Ectopic beats? _____   **No**

What kind? _____

Conclusion: _____   **AV Wenckebach**

This second-degree AV block, type I (Wenckebach), has 3.2 and 2:1 AV conduction. The sinus P waves occur at regular intervals. The PR interval lengthens, and there are nonconducted beats.

Tracing 4-13

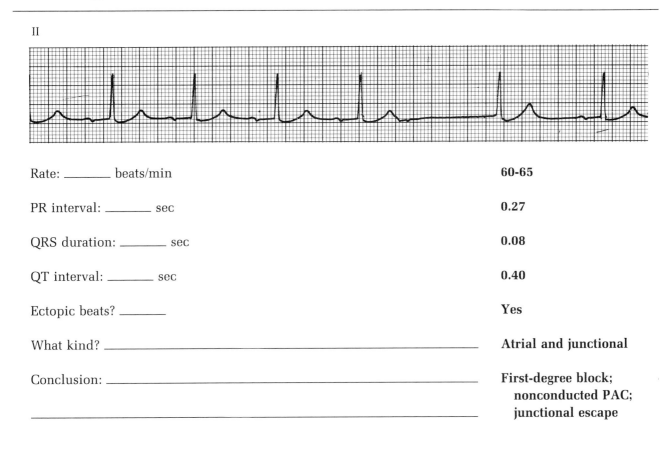

Rate: _____ beats/min   **60-65**

PR interval: _____ sec   **0.27**

QRS duration: _____ sec   **0.08**

QT interval: _____ sec   **0.40**

Ectopic beats? _____   **Yes**

What kind? _____   **Atrial and junctional**

Conclusion: _____ **First-degree block;**
_____   **nonconducted PAC;**
                                            junctional escape

This is a first-degree heart block with a nonconducted PAC, followed by a junctional escape beat. There is a P′ wave distorting the T preceding the pause.

Tracing 4-14

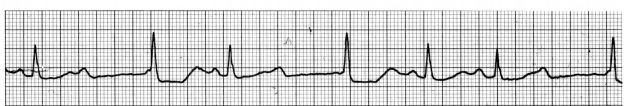

Rate: _____ beats/min   **55-60**

PR interval: _____ sec   **Varies**

QRS duration: _____ sec   **0.08**

QT interval: _____ sec   **0.64**

Ectopic beats? _____   **Yes**

What kind? _____   **Junctional**

Conclusion: _____   **AV Wenckebach;
junctional escape**

_____

The Wenckebach cycle can be seen toward the end of the tracing, where two conducted beats in a row are seen. Note the slightly different morphology of the junctional escape beats. They are taller than the sinus-conducted beats; in addition, they are distorted by a sinus P wave that occurs at the same time, causing the complex to look as though it has a delta wave.

If your diagnosis was incorrect, review the following steps. Start from the beginning and walk out the P waves. They are right on time, hiding in Rs and Ts. Then begin to establish conduction. Right away you know that there *is* conduction, because of the irregularity of the ventricular rhythm. An idiojunctional rhythm would be absolutely regular. Note that three PR intervals are the same. They are sinus-conducted beats. The two conducted beats in a row at the end of the tracing confirm the diagnosis. The junctional escape beats are easily spotted not only because they follow the long pause but also because they are slightly different in morphology.

Tracing 4-15

II

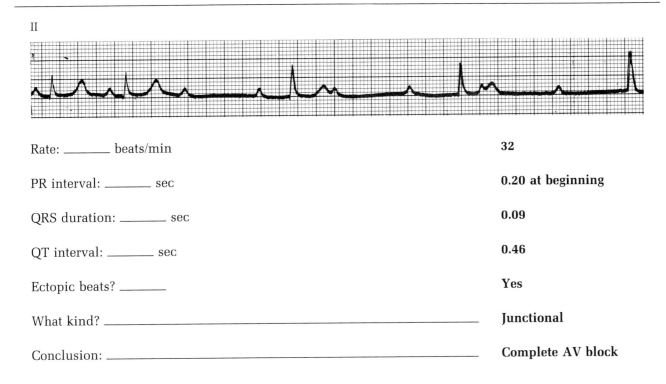

Rate: _____ beats/min	**32**
PR interval: _____ sec	**0.20 at beginning**
QRS duration: _____ sec	**0.09**
QT interval: _____ sec	**0.46**
Ectopic beats? _____	**Yes**
What kind? _____	**Junctional**
Conclusion: _____	**Complete AV block**

Here you see the onset of complete heart block. There is not even an increment in PR interval preceding the block. The patient is suddenly in third-degree heart block. His heart rate drops from 72 to 32 beats/min in a moment. Such an abrupt transition is usually accompanied by Adams-Stokes syndrome.

The escape rhythm accompanying the complete heart block is idiojunctional because the complexes are only slightly different in morphology from the sinus-conducted beats. The last ventricular complex on the tracing is broadened because there is a P wave hidden it it.

You may have thought that this patient went into Wenckebach because of the lengthening PR intervals. Remember that when there are two P waves between R waves, as seen here, all of the PR intervals have to be exactly the same in order to label the condition second-degree heart block. When the conduction ratio is 2:1, whether there is Wenckebach or type II second-degree heart block, the PR intervals will all be the same. The PR intervals lengthen in Wenckebach *only when there are two conducted beats in a row.*

Tracing 4-16

V₁

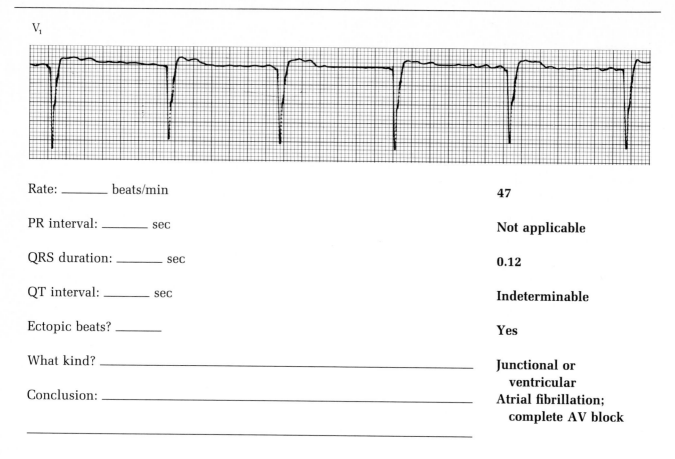

Rate: _____ beats/min

PR interval: _____ sec

QRS duration: _____ sec

QT interval: _____ sec

Ectopic beats? _____

What kind? _____

Conclusion: _____

_____

47

Not applicable

0.12

Indeterminable

Yes

Junctional or ventricular

Atrial fibrillation; complete AV block

The atrial fibrillatory line is seen through the tracing. In atrial fibrillation you expect to encounter an irregular ventricular response. Regularity of the ventricular response indicates that the ventricles are not influenced by the erratic atrial activity because there is a block. In such a case there will be either an idiojunctional pacemaker or an idioventricular one. The rate here indicates an idiojunctional pacemaker. However, the QRS is broad, indicating either bundle-branch block or an accelerated idioventricular pacemaker.

Digitalis is given to patients with atrial fibrillation to slow down the ventricular rate, which usually exceeds 100 beats/min. This drug will accomplish this by lengthening the refractory period in the AV node. If too much digitalis is given, heart block will ensue, the first sign of which is regularization. Complete block will be manifested by absolute regularity or by group beating, which is the result of Wenchebach exit block from the junctional pacemaker.

Tracing 4-17

II

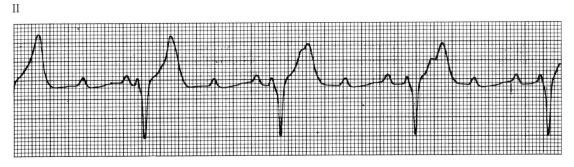

Rate: _____ beats/min

PR interval: _____ sec

QRS duration: _____ sec

QT interval: _____ sec

Ectopic beats? _____

What kind? _____

Conclusion: _____

40

Not applicable

0.16

0.56

Yes

Ventricular

Complete AV block

This is a complete heart block with a sinus tachycardia of 125 beats/min and an idioventricular rate of 40 beats/min.

If you mistook this for 2:1 block, note that the PR intervals are all of different lengths, and a closer examination of the T waves reveals hidden P waves. Mark off the first two visible P waves, and walk out the atrial rhythm. You will find the sinus rhythm regular, with P waves hidden in T waves and distorting ST segments.

Tracing 4-18

V_1

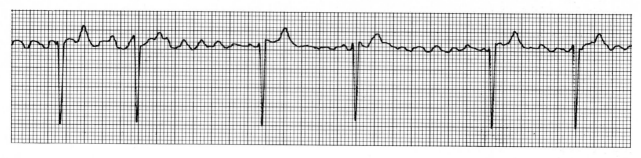

Rate: _____ beats/min   **60**

PR interval: _____ sec   **Not applicable**

QRS duration: _____ sec   **0.08**

QT interval: _____ sec   **Indeterminable**

Ectopic beats? _____   **Uncertain**

What kind? _____

Conclusion: _____   **Atrial fibrillation;
                                                      bradycardia**

   The bradycardia in this atrial fibrillation should alert you to the possibility of digitalis excess. Narrow ventricular complexes during atrial fibrillation may be conducted from the fibrillating atria, or they may be junctional beats.

Tracing 4-19

V₁

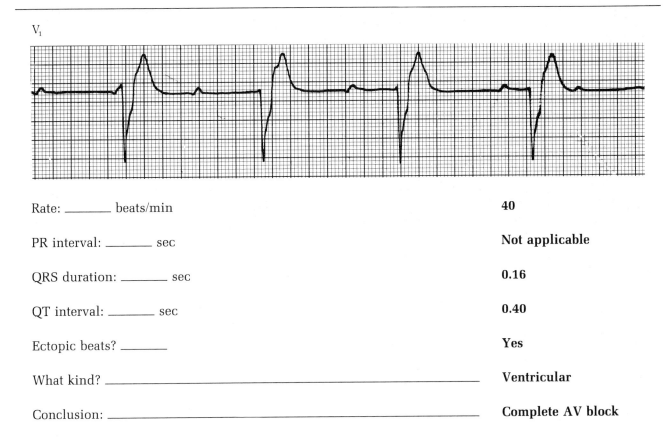

Rate: _____ beats/min   **40**

PR interval: _____ sec   **Not applicable**

QRS duration: _____ sec   **0.16**

QT interval: _____ sec   **0.40**

Ectopic beats? _____   **Yes**

What kind? _____   **Ventricular**

Conclusion: _____   **Complete AV block**

This is a complete heart block with a sinus rate of approximately 70 beats/min and a slight sinus arrhythmia. The ventricular rhythm is regular at 40 beats/min. The rate of the ventricular beats may indicate a pacemaker below the branching portion of the bundle of His (broad QRS). An idio-junctional pacemaker with bundle-branch block is also a possibility.

Almost every other P wave is hidden in the QRS-T complex. However, the first two P waves are visible and can help you find the others. The second P wave causes the first QRS to look as though it begins with a broad r wave.

Tracing 4-20

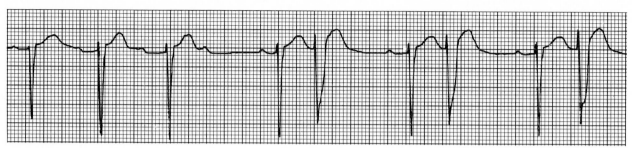

Rate: _____ beats/min   **90**

PR interval: _____ sec   **Varies**

QRS duration: _____ sec   **0.09**

QT interval: _____ sec   **0.34**

Ectopic beats? _____ sec   **Yes**

What kind? _____   **Ventricular**

Conclusion: _____   **AV Wenckebach;**
                                                           ventricular bigeminy
_____

Except for the tell-tale sign at the beginning of this tracing, the bige-minal PVCs would have masked the presence of type I second-degree heart block. Notice the lengthening PR intervals and the dropped beat (first four P waves).

Tracing 4-21

II

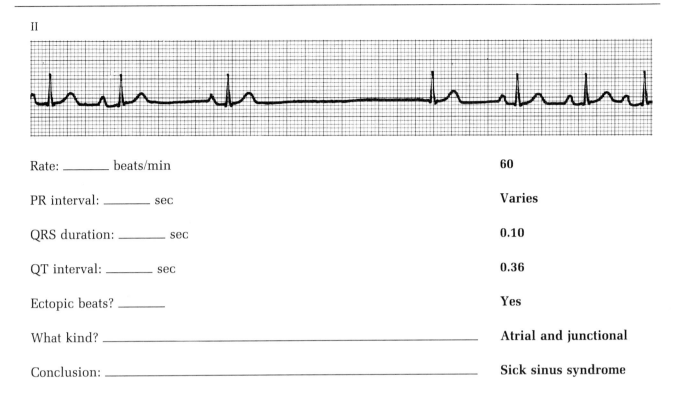

Rate: _____ beats/min   **60**

PR interval: _____ sec   **Varies**

QRS duration: _____ sec   **0.10**

QT interval: _____ sec   **0.36**

Ectopic beats? _____   **Yes**

What kind? _____   **Atrial and junctional**

Conclusion: _____   **Sick sinus syndrome**

This tracing reflects SA block and qualifies as a sick sinus syndrome, since an escape beat fails to appear and the sinus rate after the long pause jumps to 90 beats/min. There is an atrial escape beat, a junctional escape beat, and an underlying second-degree heart block (Wenckebach).

There are two normal sinus beats at the beginning of the tracing, followed by a period of sinus inactivity. This is terminated by the atrial escape beat (the third P wave). It is of different morphology from the sinus P waves and demonstrates the latent pacemaker function of the atrial specialized conductive system. Another period of sinus exit block ensues. This time it is terminated by a junctional escape beat.

The hemodynamic effects of such long pauses in rhythm can be very profound and damaging. Patients with sick sinus syndrome may not respond favorably to atropine and may require a pacemaker.

5
ATRIOVENTRICULAR DISSOCIATION

- ☐ Sinus bradycardia with junctional escape
- ☐ SA block with junctional escape
- ☐ Accelerated idiojunctional rhythm
- ☐ Accelerated idioventricular rhythm
- ☐ Junctional tachycardia
- ☐ Second-degree AV block with junctional escape
- ☐ Second-degree AV block with an accelerated idiojunctional rhythm
- ☐ Third-degree AV block
- ☐ Ventricular tachycardia
- ☐ Combinations of the above
- ☐ Isorhythmic AV dissociation

Causes of AV dissociation

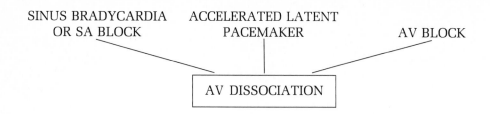

SINUS BRADYCARDIA
OR SA BLOCK   ACCELERATED LATENT
PACEMAKER   AV BLOCK

AV DISSOCIATION

AV dissociation is always _____ to another condition.   **secondary**

AV dissociation exists when the atria are being paced by one focus and the   **ventricles**
_____ by another.

VARIETIES OF AV DISSOCIATION

Sinus bradycardia with junctional escape
SA block with junctional escape
Accelerated idiojunctional rhythm
Accelerated idioventricular rhythm
Junctional tachycardia
Second-degree AV block with junctional escape
Second-degree AV block with an accelerated idiojunctional rhythm
Third-degree AV block
Ventricular tachycardia
Combinations of the above

VARIATIONS DEPEND ON

Rate and/or regularity of the two pacemakers
Presence and degree of anterograde and/or retrograde block

Tracing 5-1

II

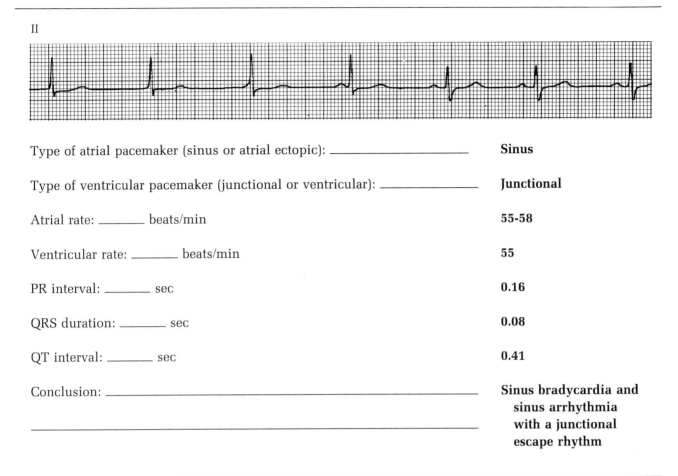

Type of atrial pacemaker (sinus or atrial ectopic): _____ **Sinus**

Type of ventricular pacemaker (junctional or ventricular): _____ **Junctional**

Atrial rate: _____ beats/min **55-58**

Ventricular rate: _____ beats/min **55**

PR interval: _____ sec **0.16**

QRS duration: _____ sec **0.08**

QT interval: _____ sec **0.41**

Conclusion: _____ **Sinus bradycardia and
sinus arrhythmia
with a junctional
escape rhythm**
_____

In this tracing the rate of the sinus node drops below that of the AV junction, so that the junctional pacemaker escapes and protects the ventricles from an excessively slow rate. At the onset of this tracing the junctional focus is in command of the ventricles and the patient has lost the benefit of the atrial kick, which deprives him of at least 20% of the cardiac output. The sinus P wave can be seen speeding up and emerging from the third complex. By the fourth complex it is in front of the ventricular complex but not far enough in front to capture, since this patient's PR interval is 0.16 sec and the junctional focus fires before that time. The fifth complex is a sinus-conducted beat. Note the slight difference in morphology between the junctional beats and the sinus-conducted ones.

The term "AV dissociation" is a symptom; it is not a diagnosis, and one must take care to determine the cause.

Tracing 5-2

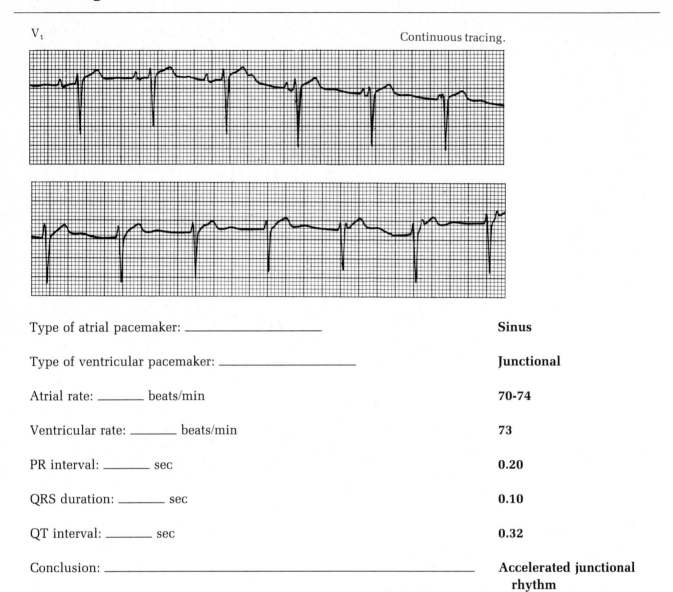

V₁   Continuous tracing.

Type of atrial pacemaker: _____	**Sinus**
Type of ventricular pacemaker: _____	**Junctional**
Atrial rate: _____ beats/min	**70-74**
Ventricular rate: _____ beats/min	**73**
PR interval: _____ sec	**0.20**
QRS duration: _____ sec	**0.10**
QT interval: _____ sec	**0.32**
Conclusion: _____	**Accelerated junctional rhythm**

This can also be called an accelerated idiojunctional rhythm, since there is no retrograde conduction to the atria, which are under the control of the sinus node. The result is AV dissociation. However, the most important consideration is the junctional rate of 73 beats/min. This is not a normal escape rate for the junction and is the result of enhanced automaticity. Once the rate reaches 100 beats/min the condition is called junctional tachycardia. This arrhythmia is commonly secondary to digitalis toxicity.

Tracing 5-3

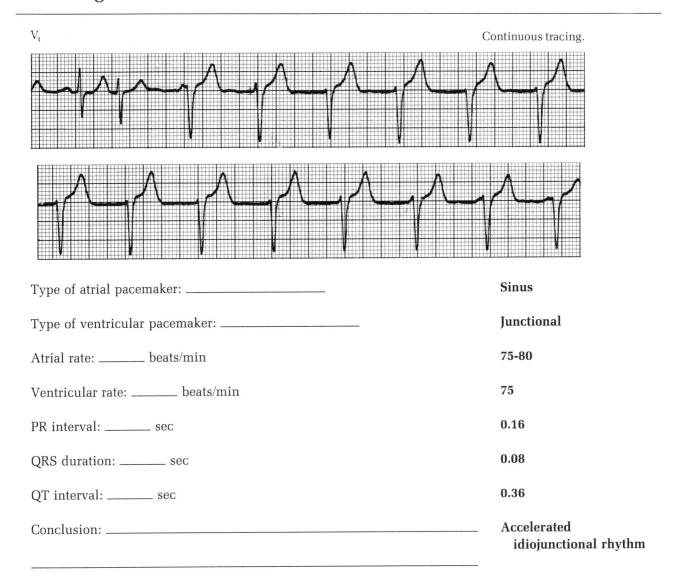

Type of atrial pacemaker: _____	**Sinus**
Type of ventricular pacemaker: _____	**Junctional**
Atrial rate: _____ beats/min	**75-80**
Ventricular rate: _____ beats/min	**75**
PR interval: _____ sec	**0.16**
QRS duration: _____ sec	**0.08**
QT interval: _____ sec	**0.36**
Conclusion: _____	**Accelerated idiojunctional rhythm**

This accelerated idiojunctional rhythm was unmasked by the pause following a PAC. The first beat is sinus conducted; it is followed by a PAC (in the T). The pause following the PAC is not excessive, but it is about 0.08 sec longer than that of the sinus cycle, giving us a chance to see the accelerated junctional focus, which, along with the PAC, may be a manifestation of digitalis toxicity. Note the different and yet not abnormal shape of the junctional complex. In the bottom half of this strip the P wave begins to distort the beginning of the QRS.

Tracing 5-4

II

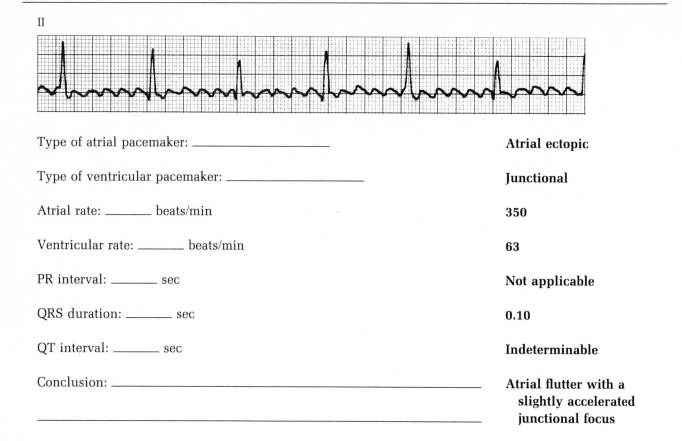

Type of atrial pacemaker: _____   **Atrial ectopic**

Type of ventricular pacemaker: _____   **Junctional**

Atrial rate: _____ beats/min   **350**

Ventricular rate: _____ beats/min   **63**

PR interval: _____ sec   **Not applicable**

QRS duration: _____ sec   **0.10**

QT interval: _____ sec   **Indeterminable**

Conclusion: _____   **Atrial flutter with a**
_____   **slightly accelerated**
                                                         junctional focus

The typical sawtooth pattern of atrial flutter is seen throughout the strip. However, there is no constant relationship between the flutter waves and the QRS complex. This is a sign of AV dissociation or heart block coexisting with the atrial flutter. It is most probably AV dissociation with occasional conduction, since the ventricular rhythm is not absolutely regular. This means that the atria are beating at a rate of 350 beats/min but that only an occasional impulse is being conducted to the ventricles, which are mainly under the control of an independent junctional focus with a rate of 63 beats/min.

Tracing 5-5

V₁

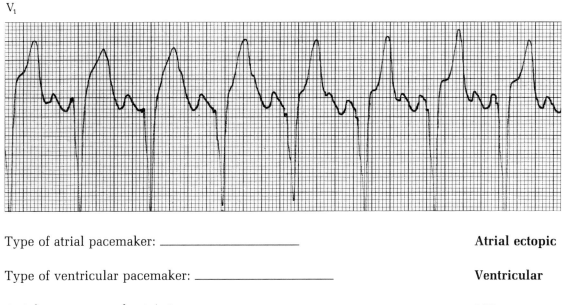

Type of atrial pacemaker: _____   **Atrial ectopic**

Type of ventricular pacemaker: _____   **Ventricular**

Atrial rate: _____ beats/min   **300**

Ventricular rate: _____ beats/min   **78**

PR interval: _____ sec   **Not applicable**

QRS duration: _____ sec   **0.12**

QT interval: _____ sec   **0.44**

Conclusion: _____   **Atrial flutter with**
_____   **an accelerated**
idioventricular
rhythm

Here again, as in the previous tracing, is AV dissociation in the presence of atrial flutter. Note the changing relationship between the flutter waves and the ventricular complex. This, the width of the ventricular complexes, and the regularity of the ventricular rhythm indicate that the ventricular rhythm is independent of the atrial rhythm and that the ventricular ectopic focus is below the branching portion of the bundle of His.

Tracing 5-6

V$_1$

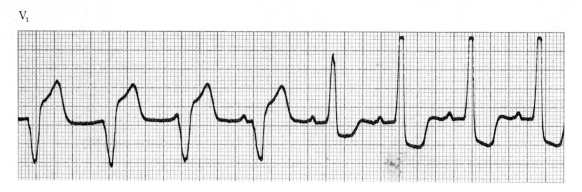

Type of atrial pacemaker: _____   **Sinus**

Type of ventricular pacemaker: _____   **Ventricular**

Atrial rate: _____ beats/min   **75-80**

Ventricular rate: _____ beats/min   **76**

PR interval: _____ sec   **0.22**

QRS duration: _____ sec   **0.12**

QT interval: _____ sec   **0.49**

Conclusion: _____

_____   **Accelerated idioventricular rhythm**

The ventricular ectopic focus can be seen beating at the beginning of the tracing. It has an accelerated rate of 76 and dominates the ventricles as long as the sinus node is slower. Toward the middle of the tracing you will notice the P wave begin to emerge from the ventricular ectopic beat as the rate of sinus node speeds up from 75 to 80. There is one fusion beat (the fifth) before the sinus node is in complete control of the ventricles.

Tracing 5-7

II

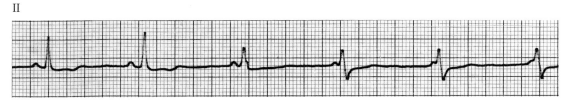

Type of atrial pacemaker: _____   **Sinus**

Type of ventricular pacemaker: _____   **Ventricular**

Atrial rate: _____ beats/min   **55**

Ventricular rate: _____ beats/min   **56**

PR interval: _____ sec   **0.14**

QRS duration: _____ sec   **0.08**

QT interval: _____ sec   **0.40**

Conclusion: _____   **Accelerated**
_____   **idioventricular rhythm and sinus bradycardia**

The sinus bradycardia can be seen at the beginning of the tracing. The third beat is a fusion complex caused by the simultaneous firing of the ventricular ectopic focus and activation of the ventricles by the sinus impulse. Notice how the sinus P wave distorts the ventricular ectopic complex. A rate of 56 would be considered an escape rhythm if the focus were in the AV junction instead of the ventricles. The fusion beat proves the ventricular origin of the ectopic rhythm; plus there is the fact that the QRS complex of the ectopic rhythm is broad.

Tracing 5-8

II

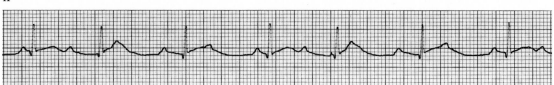

Type of atrial pacemaker: _____	**Sinus**
Type of ventricular pacemaker: _____	**Junctional**
Atrial rate: _____ beats/min	**114**
Ventricular rate: _____ beats/min	**65**
PR interval: _____ sec	**0.36**
QRS duration: _____ sec	**0.06**
QT interval: _____ sec	**0.48**
Conclusion: _____ _____	**Accelerated idiojunctional rhythm and sinus tachycardia**

There are two sinus-conducted beats in this tracing. Can you find them? They are recognized because there is a shorter cycle preceding them and they interrupt the regular rhythm of the junctional focus. They are the second and the fifth beats.

In this tracing the accelerated junctional focus dominates the ventricles until the sinus P wave lands far enough away from the preceding R wave to find a nonrefractory route into the ventricles. When it would seem that the P wave should be able to conduct into the ventricles (third and fourth complexes) and yet does not, there are two factors to consider: (1) the P wave in the preceding T may have partially penetrated the AV junction (concealed conduction), leaving it refractory to the next beat, and (2) there may be some degree of AV block, so that the accelerated junctional focus fires before the sinus impulse can negotiate the AV node.

In this tracing there are two signs of digitalis toxicity: accelerated idiojunctional rhythm and AV block.

Tracing 5-9

II

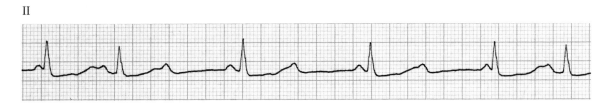

Type of atrial pacemaker: _____	**Sinus**
Type of ventricular pacemaker: _____	**Junctional**
Atrial rate: _____ beats/min	**88**
Ventricular rate: _____ beats/min	**44**
PR interval: _____ sec	**0.22**
QRS duration: _____ sec	**0.08**
QT interval: _____ sec	**0.68**
Conclusion: _____	**AV block (some degree)**
_____	**with a junctional escape rhythm**

This AV dissociation is probably caused by the excessively long QT interval, which reflects a long refractory period. There are some P waves that are certainly in a position to conduct; that is, they are far enough away from the preceding R wave, but fall on the T. Then before the next sinus P wave has a chance to conduct, there is a junctional escape beat.

As in the last tracing, there are two sinus-conducted beats. Find them by the same rules. Look for a shortening of the cycle length. The two P waves that are conducted may represent supernormal conduction, in which conduction is better than expected because activiation occurs at a very precise spot at the end of the T wave, when the heart is almost completely repolarized.

Tracing 5-10

II

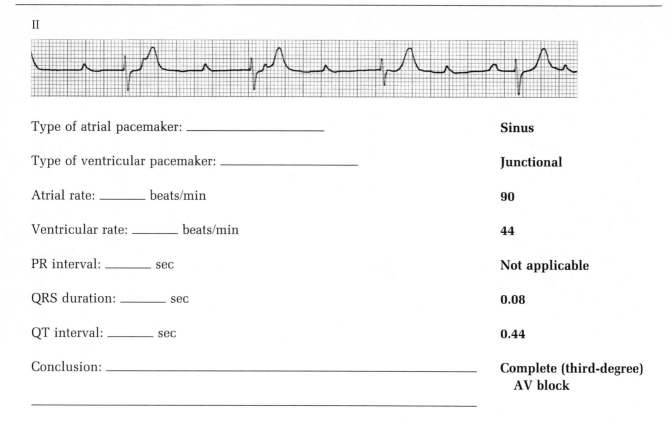

Type of atrial pacemaker: _____   **Sinus**

Type of ventricular pacemaker: _____   **Junctional**

Atrial rate: _____ beats/min   **90**

Ventricular rate: _____ beats/min   **44**

PR interval: _____ sec   **Not applicable**

QRS duration: _____ sec   **0.08**

QT interval: _____ sec   **0.44**

Conclusion: _____   **Complete (third-degree)**
          AV block

_____

In complete heart block there is a pathological block between the atria and the ventricles. It is physically impossible for impulses to pass, under any conditions. Because of the pathology, this type of AV dissociation is different from the previous ones seen in this chapter. In AV dissociation resulting from other causes the failure to conduct is physiological.

Tracing 5-11

II

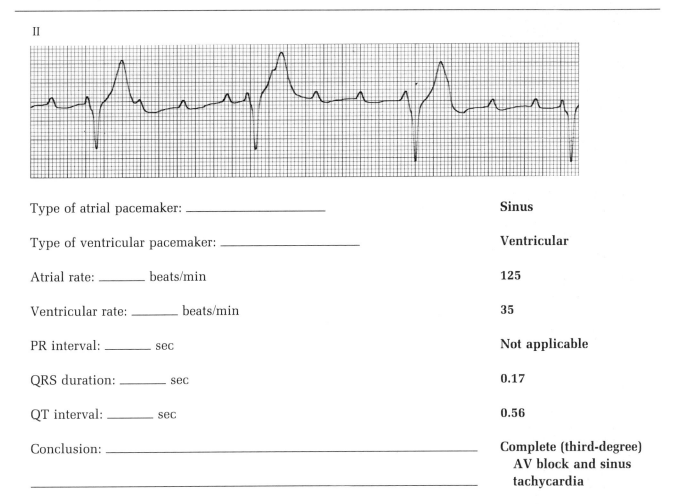

Type of atrial pacemaker: _____ **Sinus**

Type of ventricular pacemaker: _____ **Ventricular**

Atrial rate: _____ beats/min **125**

Ventricular rate: _____ beats/min **35**

PR interval: _____ sec **Not applicable**

QRS duration: _____ sec **0.17**

QT interval: _____ sec **0.56**

Conclusion: _____ **Complete (third-degree) AV block and sinus tachycardia**

_____

Here is another example of AV dissociation resulting from complete heart block. This patient had taken an overdose of digitalis. There is an idioventricular pacemaker in control of the ventricles.

Tracing 5-12

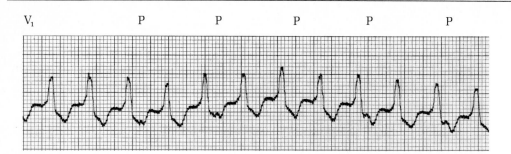

Type of atrial pacemaker: _____   **Sinus**

Type of ventricular pacemaker: _____   **Ventricular**

Atrial rate: _____ beats/min   **70**

Ventricular rate: _____ beats/min   **145**

PR interval: _____ sec   **Not applicable**

QRS duration: _____ sec   **0.12**

QT interval: _____ sec   **Indeterminable**

Conclusion: _____   **Ventricular tachycardia**

Although the signs of AV dissociation in ventricular tachycardia (independent P waves) are not often apparent, they are proof of the ventricular origin of the tachycardia and are therefore useful in the differential diagnosis between ventricular ectopy and ventricular aberration.

When there is 1:1 or 2:1 retrograde activation of the atria, ventricular tachycardia exists without AV dissociation. Such is the case in the tracing below, where you will notice 2:1 retrograde conduction.

II

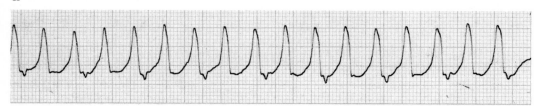

6
LADDERGRAMS

- [ ] **PACs**
- [ ] **AV block**
- [ ] **AV reciprocating mechanisms**
- [ ] **PVCs**
- [ ] **Fusion beats**

Laddergrams defined

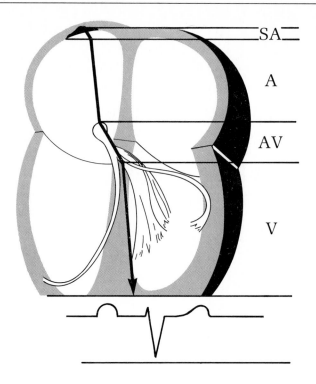

Laddergrams (Lewis diagrams) are stick figures illustrating the sequence of AV conduction.

The tiers of the graph show SA conduction (when there is an SA conduction problem) and conduction through the _____, _____ _____, and _____.   **atria; AV junction; ventricles**

The leading point on the diagram indicates the _____.   **pacemaker**

The slant of the line in the AV tier indicates the AV _____ time.   **conduction**

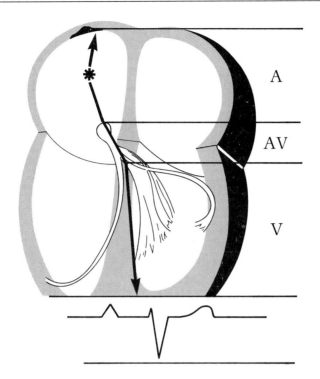

To illustrate a PAC with normal ventricular conduction, the leading point of the stick figure is placed within the _____ tier.

atrial

AV block

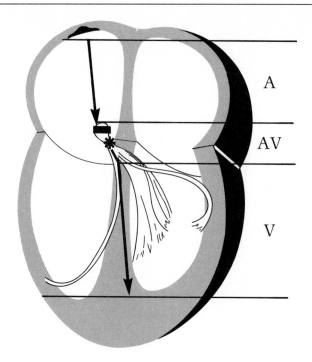

A

AV

V

To illustrate complete AV block, a _____ impulse is drawn
in the atrial tier and a pacemaker is indicated within the AV
_____.

sinus

junction

AV nodal reentry (PSVT)

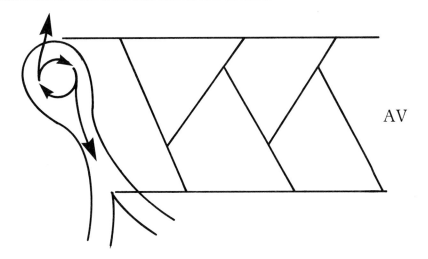

AV

In order to illustrate the _____ mechanism of PSVT, reflecting lines are drawn in the _____ tier.

reciprocating
AV

Tracing 6-1

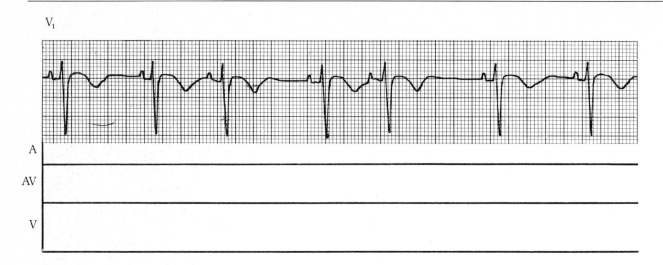

Begin your laddergram by filling in the P waves in the A tier and then the ventricular complexes in the V tier. Compare what you have done with the laddergram below. Notice that since the laddergram depicts a *sequence* of events, the PACs will be indicated by placing a leading point in the middle of the A tier instead of at the top of it as is done for the sinus P waves. Now simply fill in AV conduction by drawing a straight line from the end of the P wave line to the top of the QRS line.

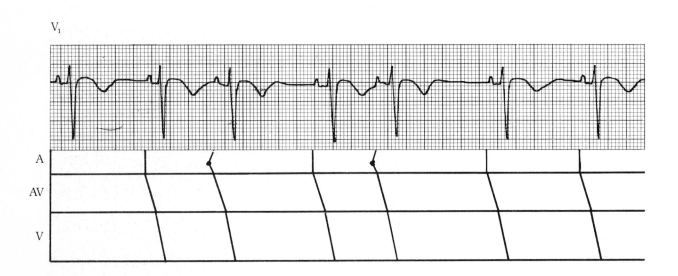

Tracing 6-2

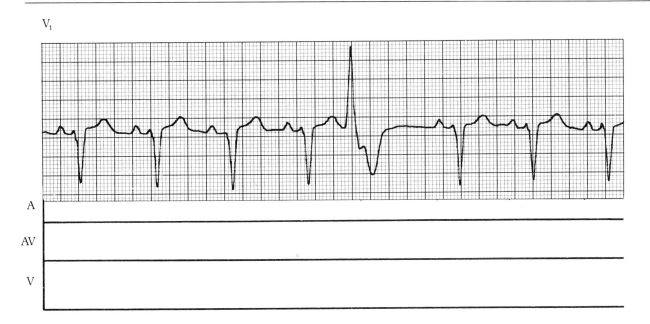

Begin your laddergram as before, and you will easily find the hidden sinus P wave occurring right on time. It is in the T wave of the ectopic beat.

The ventricular ectopic complex is illustrated by placing the leading point at the bottom of the V tier at a spot directly below where the PVC begins. The V line will then proceed upward in this tier, slanting toward the top of the tier at a spot directly below where the PVC ends. Normally conducted ventricular complexes are illustrated this way, too, but the slant is in the opposite direction, that is, beginning at the top of the V tier and ending at the bottom. The V line will give you some idea of intraventricular conduction time because it is slanted.

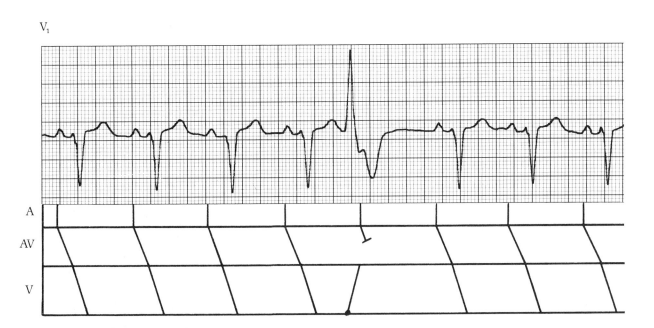

Tracing 6-3

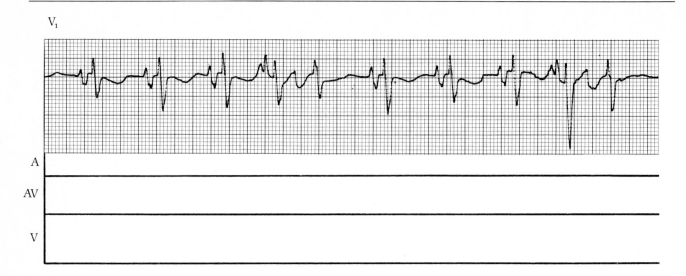

V₁

This is a more complicated mechanism to illustrate, since there are an atrial echo and a ventricular reciprocal beat. However, the laddergram is the most useful tool to explain this mechanism.

Begin, as before, by marking the P lines in the A tier. Indicate the two PACs that are so evident. Unless you are experienced and aware of reciprocating mechanisms, you will probably not see the atrial echo beat. Just leave it for now, and draw in the ventricular lines in the V tier. Indicate AV conduction; it is immediately apparent that there is a ventricular complex with no origin. You can find the atrial echo beat in the T wave preceding the complex in question. The PAC has caused dissociation within the AV node, passing antegradely to capture the ventricles and then retrogradely to recapture the atria and back down again to the ventricles. The laddergram depicts this mechanism well. The PAC at the end of the tracing is conducted with aberrancy.

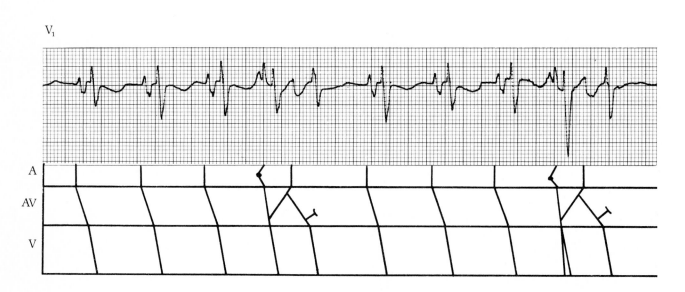

V₁

Tracing 6-4

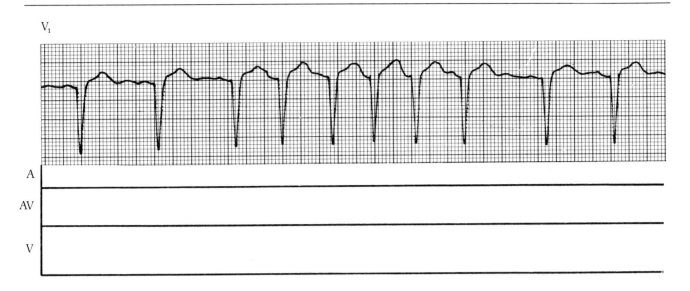

Here is another reciprocating mechanism. See if you can construct the laddergram, and then compare yours with the one below.

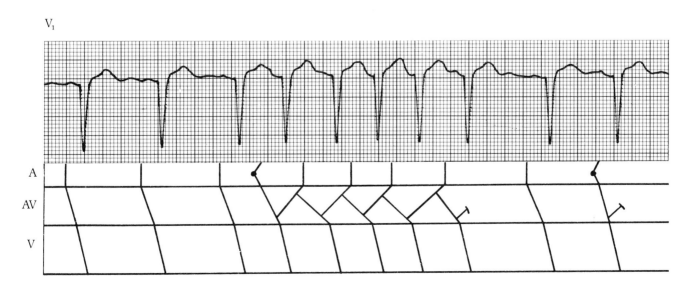

Tracing 6-5

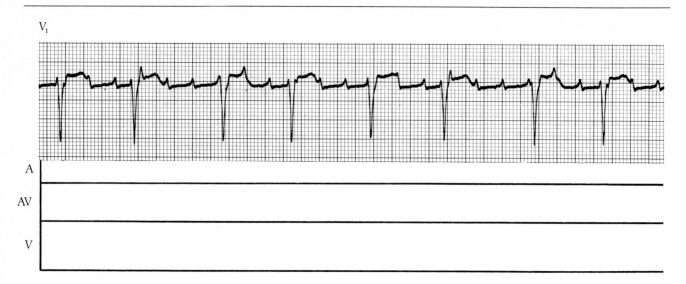

This is atrial flutter as seen in V_1. When the P'-R interval alternates as it does here, there is a Wenckebach conduction mechanism. Draw in the P' waves. Since all are ectopic, simply draw them as you would sinus P waves. Their rate alone will indicate ectopy. Now draw in the ventricular complexes, and see if you can establish the right AV conduction lines, keeping in mind a Wenckebach type of conduction. Compare your ladder-gram with the one below.

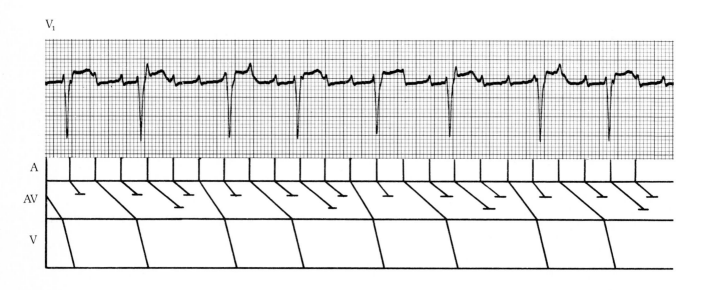

Tracing 6-6

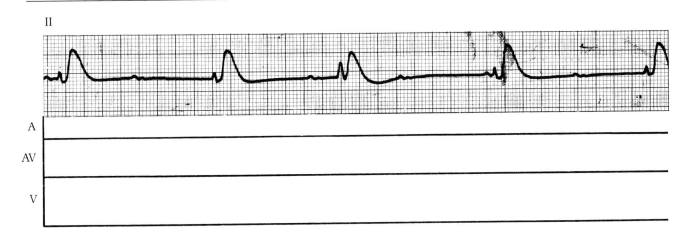

In this exercise mark in the P waves that you see. If you keep in mind the normal behavior of the sinus node, you will find the hidden ones. Draw in the ventricular complexes. They are very low in amplitude with very tall T waves. Draw the AV conduction lines, remembering the rule that when the PR intervals are all different, the RR intervals must all be equal for the condition to be complete heart block. If there is a QRS out of step, it will be "pulled in" (early, conducted). Compare your laddergram with the one below. This is a high-grade second-degree heart block. Notice that the conducted beat is of slightly different morphology.

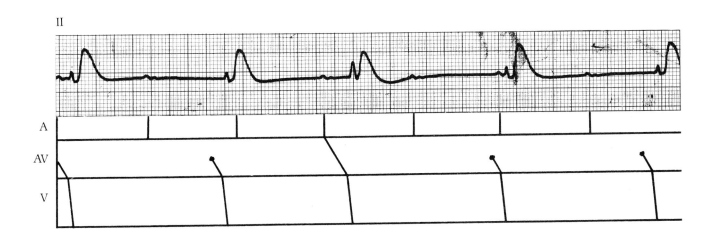

Tracing 6-7

II

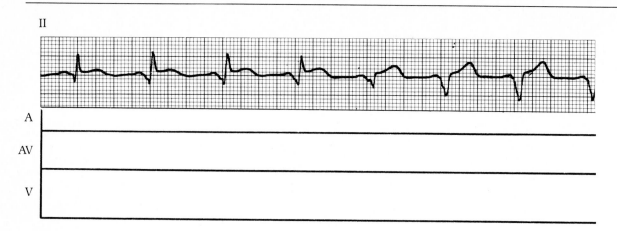

The sinus rate in this tracing is 74 beats/min. There is an accelerated idioventricular focus competing at a rate of 75. The ventricular ectopic focus can be seen manifesting itself in the second complex. This complex and the four after it are fusion beats, with the ventricular ectopic focus capturing the ventricles more completely each time until finally it is premature enough for complete capture.

The laddergram appropriately illustrates why ventricular fusion beats seldom look just the same in a particular lead. It is because the degrees of fusion are never exactly the same.

II

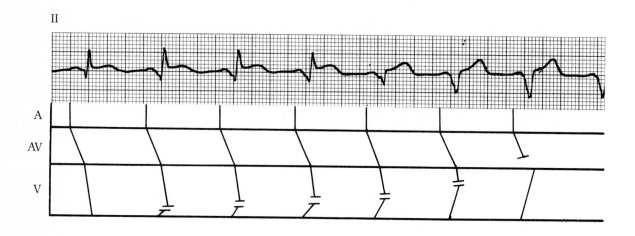

Tracing 6-8

II

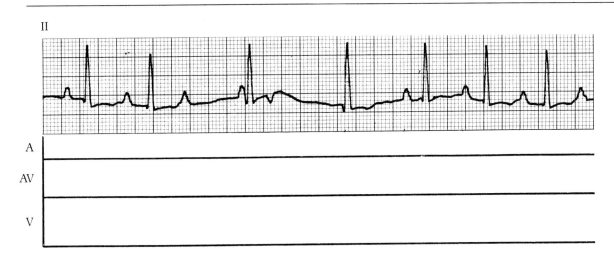

Your laddergram, properly done, will indicate that this is a type I second-degree heart block with two junctional escape beats. Compare your laddergram with the one below.

In the absence of a laddergram, the following explanation would be in order: The first two P waves are conducted with lengthening PR intervals. The third P wave is not conducted, and before the fourth P wave has a chance to conduct, there is a junctional escape beat with retrograde atrial conduction. The next complex represents a junctional escape mechanism with simultaneous antegrade and retrograde conduction. After this, the sinus node resumes its role as pacemaker, and impulses are once again conducted with increasing PR intervals. This is an atypical Wenckebach in that the second PR interval does not have the greatest increment nor is there a shortening of the RR interval.

II

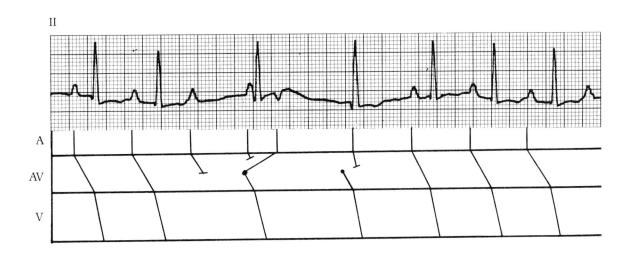

Tracing 6-9

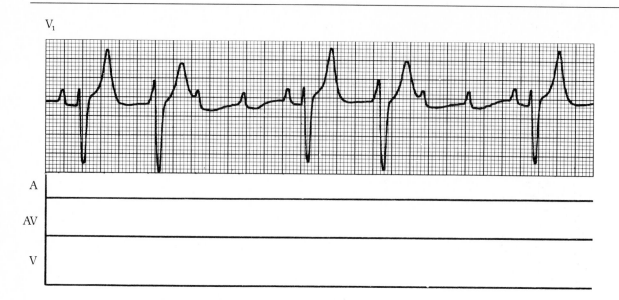

Here is one case in which a laddergram is necessary in order to establish the sequence of AV conduction. As you mark off the P waves in the A tier, you are reminded that the sinus node is expected to beat at regular intervals. Thus you find P waves hidden in T waves and r waves. When it is time to draw the lines in the AV tier, you note that the second beat of the pairs is not really as aberrant as it looks, since a P wave distorts it. It is a supraventricular beat conducted from the P in the preceding T—a Wenckebach (5:2) conduction pattern. There is an underlying sinus tachycardia.

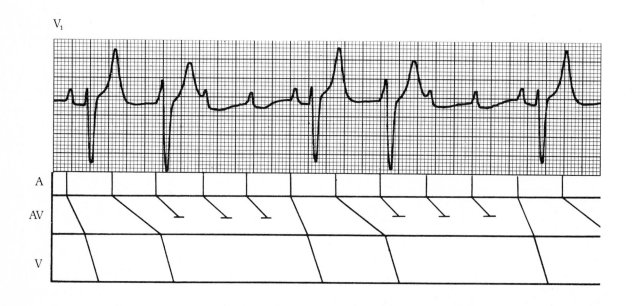

Tracing 6-10

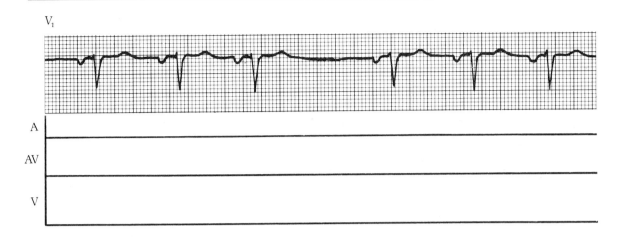

Aside from a lengthy explanation, a laddergram is probably the only clear way to illustrate the mechanism of this arrhythmia, although if you know the rules governing a sinus rhythm, you can easily diagnose this arrhythmia without a laddergram. One rule is as follows: shortening PP intervals and a pause that is less than twice the shortest cycle indicate a Wenckebach mechanism. This is a sinus node Wenckebach.

In order to build the laddergram, count the number of cycles in a group, including the dropped beat (a missing P in this case). Now divide this number (4) into the total length of the Wenckebach cycle (320 msec), and you will come up with the interval between the firing of each sinus node beat (80 msec). Start with the first P wave of a group and estimate a small amount of time for the sinus impulse to reach the atria. From this point walk out on the laddergram the sinus rhythm at the intervals you have calculated. This requires an additional tier at the top for SA activity. Draw in the P waves in the A tier. Draw a line from the point of sinus firing to the atrial line. The conduction time will be seen to increase each time until a beat is not conducted at all.

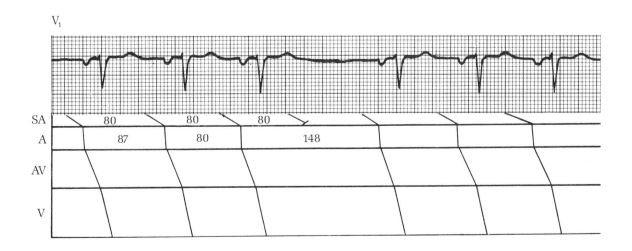

Tracing 6-11

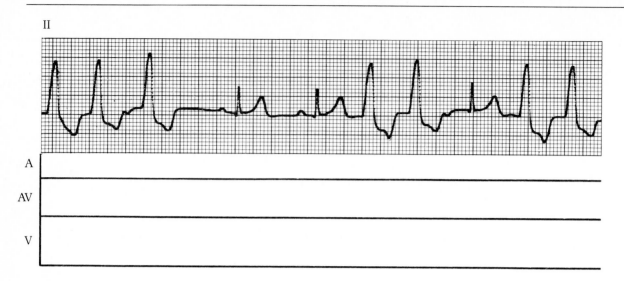

This is an interesting arrhythmia that might be missed without a laddergram. The first clue comes when you begin to mark off the P waves in the A tier. There are P waves after each PVC. The laddergram helps you to note that they are out of step with the sinus rhythm and therefore are retrograde P′ waves. Retrograde conduction time is seen to lengthen, and in the third PVC on the tracing retrograde conduction is blocked completely (a retrograde Wenckebach). The next time it happens there is a reciprocal beat; that is, the second retrograde P′ in the next set of PVCs travels back down the AV junction to recapture the ventricles.

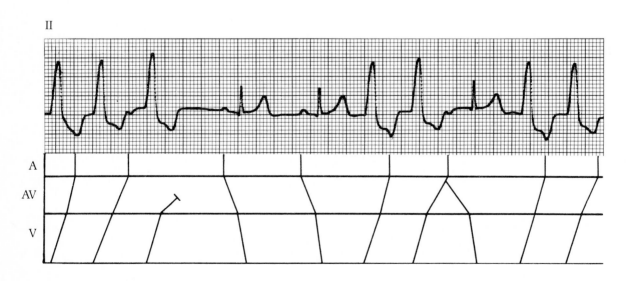

Tracing 6-12

II

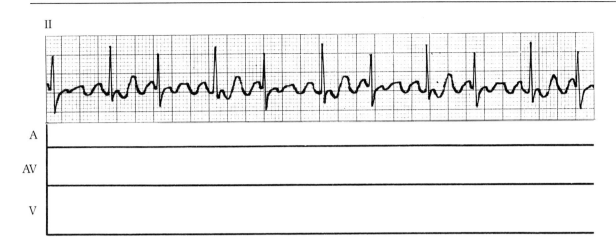

You will recognize the sawtooth pattern of atrial flutter quite readily in this tracing. The bigeminal rhythm, however, represents a more complicated mechanism. There is a Wenckebach mechanism in action. This is often the explanation when there is atrial flutter with alternating AV conduction. Here we have a basic 2:1 block with the dropped beat every other cycle.

II

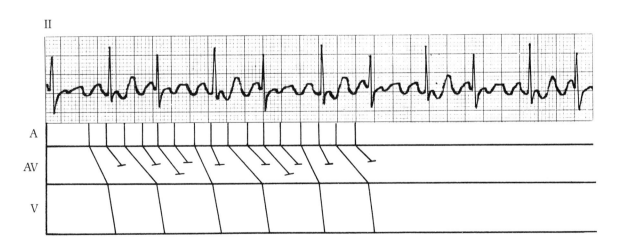

7

BUNDLE-BRANCH BLOCK

- ☐ **Normal intraventricular activation**
- ☐ **Right bundle-branch block**
- ☐ **Left bundle-branch block**
- ☐ **Left anterior hemiblock**
- ☐ **Left posterior hemiblock**

Normal intraventricular activation

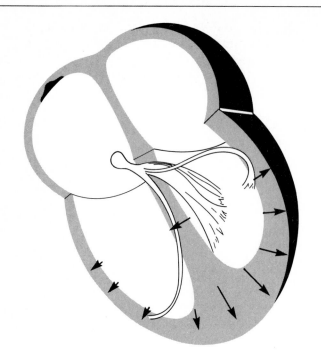

Normally both ventricles are activated at the same time, producing a narrow QRS.

Therefore, right-ventricular activation is buried in that of the _____ **left**
ventricle because the _____ ventricle is larger than the right. **left**

The normal QRS is _____. **narrow**

Since the left ventricle is larger than the right, the main current flow is
_____, toward V____ and away from V____. **leftward; V_6; V_1**

Therefore, the polarity of the QRS in V_6 is mainly _____. **positive**

V_1 is mainly _____. **negative**

Bundle-branch block

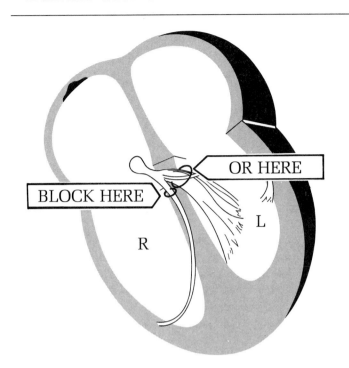

BLOCK HERE

OR HERE

R

L

The bundle branches speed the impulse to the ventricles. Therefore when a bundle branch is blocked, the ventricle served by that bundle branch is activated late and the QRS is 0.12 sec or more.

In right bundle-branch block (RBBB) the _____ ventricle is activated late.

right

In left bundle-branch block (LBBB) the _____ ventricle is activated late.

left

Right bundle-branch block

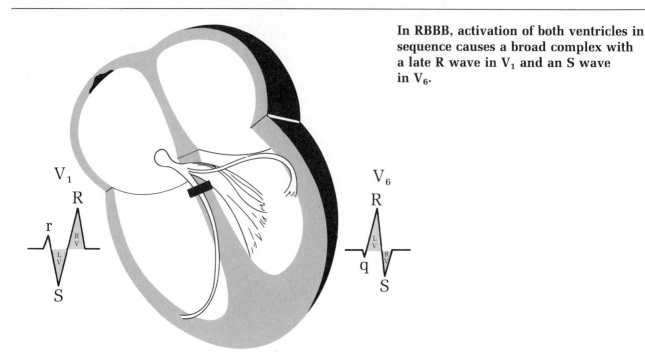

In RBBB, activation of both ventricles in sequence causes a broad complex with a late R wave in V_1 and an S wave in V_6.

Activation of both ventricles can be seen on the ECG—first the _____ ventricle and then the _____.

left
right

Therefore in V_1 there is a late _____ wave.

R

And in V_6 there is a broad _____ wave.

S

The T wave is of _____ polarity to the terminal component of the QRS.

opposite

The RBBB pattern in V₁

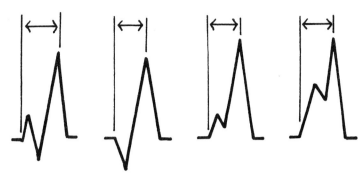

Intrinsicoid deflection (ventricular activation time) > 0.07 sec

Although the RBBB pattern in V₁ is not always triphasic (rSR′), there is always a late R wave and the complex is broad.

The ventricular activation time is measured from the beginning of the QRS to the peak of the last _____ wave.　　　　　　　　　　**R**

In RBBB the ventricular activation time is greater than _____ sec.　　　**0.07**

Left bundle-branch block

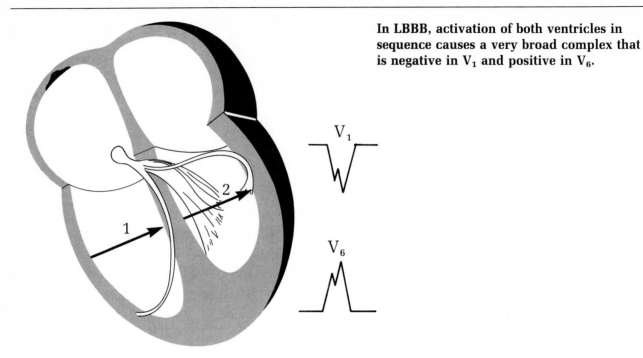

In LBBB, activation of both ventricles in sequence causes a very broad complex that is negative in V_1 and positive in V_6.

Activation of both ventricles can be seen on the ECG—first the _____ ventricle and then the _____.

right
left

Since the right ventricle is the first to be activated, the main current is _____.

leftward

This produces a _____ complex in V_1, and a _____ one in V_6.

negative; positive

The T wave is of _____ polarity to the terminal component of the QRS.

opposite

Comparison of LBBB and RBBB

V₁   V₁   **RBBB compared to LBBB in V_1.**

RBBB

LBBB

In V_1 an RBBB pattern is mainly _____.   **positive**

In V_1 an LBBB pattern is _____.   **negative**

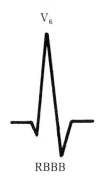   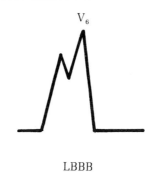   **RBBB compared to LBBB in V_6.**

In V_6 an RBBB pattern is _____.   **triphasic**

In V_6 an LBBB pattern is _____.   **positive**

Hemiblock

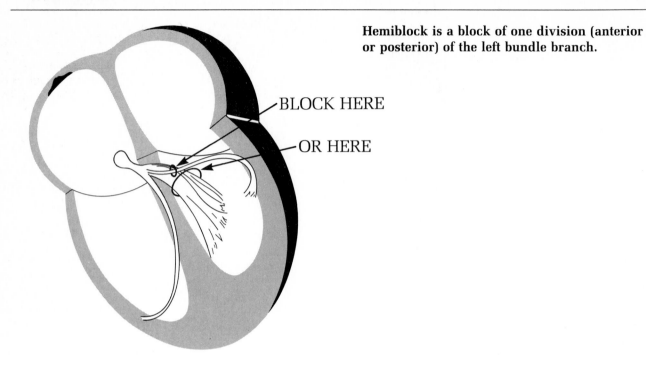

Hemiblock is a block of one division (anterior or posterior) of the left bundle branch.

BLOCK HERE

OR HERE

Hemiblock refers only to the _____ bundle branch.   **left**

Anterior hemiblock refers to a block of the _____ division   **superior**
of the left bundle branch.

Posterior hemiblock refers to a block of the _____ divi-   **inferior**
sion of the left bundle branch.

Left anterior hemiblock

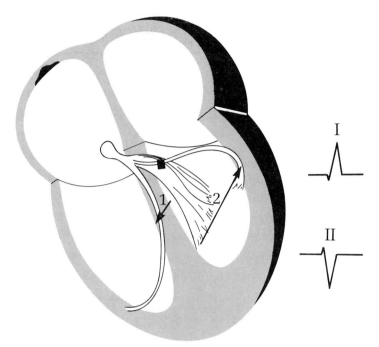

Left anterior hemiblock (LAH) causes left axis deviation.

The main current in LAH is to the _____ and superior.   **left**

This produces _____ axis deviation.   **left**

In left axis deviation the main current is _____ the positive electrode of lead I and _____ _____ the positive electrode of lead II.   **toward**   **away from**

Therefore in LAH the QRS complex is _____ in lead I and _____ in lead II.   **positive**   **negative**

Left posterior hemiblock

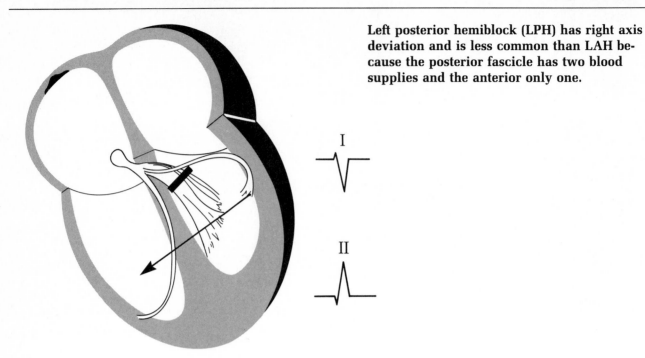

Left posterior hemiblock (LPH) has right axis deviation and is less common than LAH because the posterior fascicle has two blood supplies and the anterior only one.

The main current in LPH is to the _____ and inferior.   **right**

This produces _____ axis deviation.   **right**

In right axis deviation the main current is _____ _____   **away from**
the positive electrode of lead I and _____ the positive electrode   **toward**
of lead II.

Therefore in LAH the QRS complex is _____ in lead I and   **negative**
_____ in lead II.   **positive**

Tracing 7-1

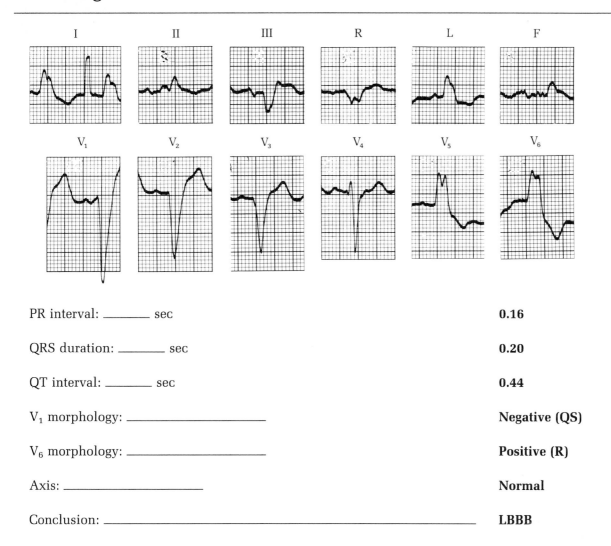

I	II	III	R	L	F

V₁	V₂	V₃	V₄	V₅	V₆

PR interval: _____ sec   **0.16**

QRS duration: _____ sec   **0.20**

QT interval: _____ sec   **0.44**

V₁ morphology: _____   **Negative (QS)**

V₆ morphology: _____   **Positive (R)**

Axis: _____   **Normal**

Conclusion: _____   **LBBB**

Certainly the most notable features of this electrocardiogram are the broad, slurred ventricular complexes that are completely negative in lead V₁. In LBBB the initial forces are altered, and ventricular depolarization commences in the septum from right to left. This is reflected in lead V₆ by absent q waves. Leads I and aV_L have a similar pattern because the positive terminals of these leads are on the left shoulder.

You are able to determine the electrical axis of the heart by noting that the ventricular complex is almost isoelectric in lead aV_F (just slightly positive in value). Since lead I has an axis that is perpendicular to the axis of aV_F, you can now almost exactly determine the heart axis by the ventricular complex in this lead. It is totally positive. Therefore the main current flow of the heart is to the left, or toward the positive terminal of lead I, and is almost perpendicular to aV$_F$ but tipped a little toward the positive terminal. The electrical axis is approximately +25°. This is a normal axis, a common finding with LBBB. A glance at leads I and II gives you the same information because positive complexes in these leads reflect a normal axis.

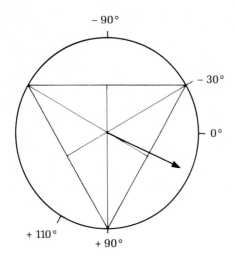

An electrical axis of +25° would be perpendicular to the axis of aV$_F$ and flowing into the positive terminal of lead I.

Tracing 7-2

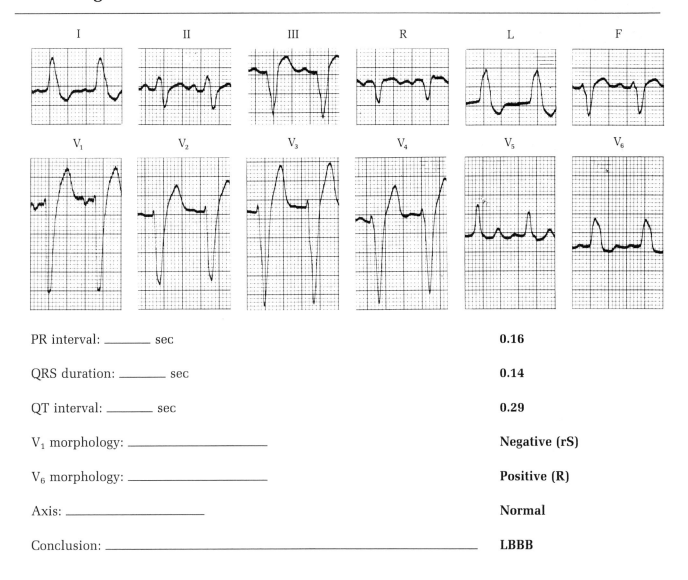

PR interval: _____ sec   **0.16**

QRS duration: _____ sec   **0.14**

QT interval: _____ sec   **0.29**

V_1 morphology: _____   **Negative (rS)**

V_6 morphology: _____   **Positive (R)**

Axis: _____   **Normal**

Conclusion: _____   **LBBB**

The broad ventricular complexes, negative in V_1, are indicative of LBBB. The absence of normal septal activation is reflected by absent q waves in leads I, aV_L, and V_6.

The electrical axis is determined by observing the equiphasic deflection in lead II and the fully positive value of aV_L, reflective of a current flowing perpendicular to the axis of lead II and full into the positive terminal of aV_L. The electrical axis of the heart is approximately $-30°$ (normal).

Note the small r wave in the right chest leads, indicating the initial activation took place in the anterior wall of the right ventricle.

When leads I and II are upright, or if one of them is equiphasic, and the axis is normal.

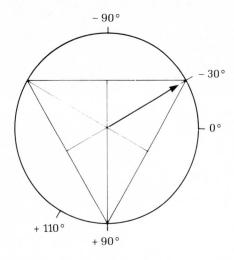

An electrical axis of −30° would be perpendicular to the axis of lead II and flowing into the positive electrode of aV_L.

Tracing 7-3

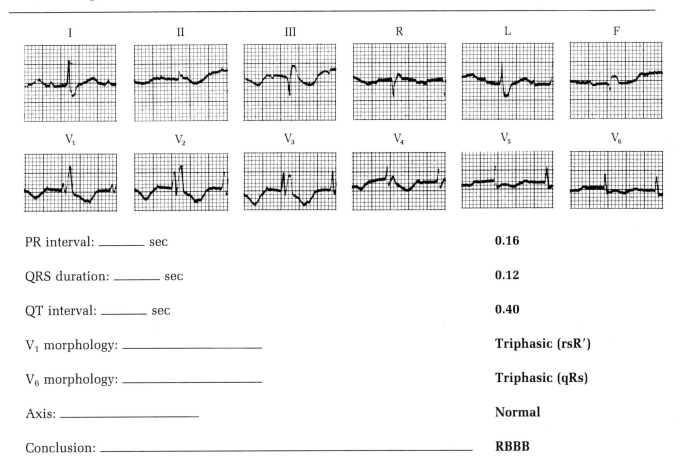

PR interval: _____ sec   **0.16**

QRS duration: _____ sec   **0.12**

QT interval: _____ sec   **0.40**

V_1 morphology: _____   **Triphasic (rsR′)**

V_6 morphology: _____   **Triphasic (qRs)**

Axis: _____   **Normal**

Conclusion: _____   **RBBB**

Notice the predominantly positive deflection (M shaped) in lead V_1. Remember that the ventricular complex in this lead is usually an rS configuration, with the small initial r wave reflecting septal depolarization and the deep S wave reflecting left-ventricular depolarization. In RBBB the initial forces and left-ventricular activation are normal. In lead V_1 this would be reflected in a small r and an S wave. However, since the right ventricle is depolarized late, this deflection would no longer be lost in the left-ventricular complex but would be quite visible as a late strong positive terminal event (R′). Leads I, aV_L, and V_6 would also reflect this late activation of the right ventricle in a broad S wave, indicating late terminal vector forces directed to the right (away from leads I and V_6).

Here again the electrical axis can be estimated simply by observing the six limb leads for an equiphasic deflection. This is found in aV_F and indicates that the main direction of current flow is perpendicular, or almost perpendicular, to the axis of this lead. Knowing the main direction of current flow, however, does not tell you whether the current flows to the right or to the left. The lead whose axis is perpendicular to that of aV_F is lead I.

Note that the ventricular complex is primarily positive in this lead, indicating that the main current flow is to the left. Since the aV$_F$ complex was not exactly equiphasic (slightly more positive than negative), we can now make a small correction toward the positive terminal of aV$_F$. The estimated axis is +10°.

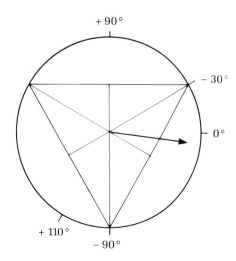

An electrical axis of +10° would be perpendicular to the axis of aV$_F$ and flowing into the positive terminal of lead I.

To check for axis shift, look at lead II and lead I. A glance will tell you whether a shift has occurred: In left axis deviation lead II will become negative, with I upright. In right axis deviation lead I will become negative, with II upright.

Tracing 7-4

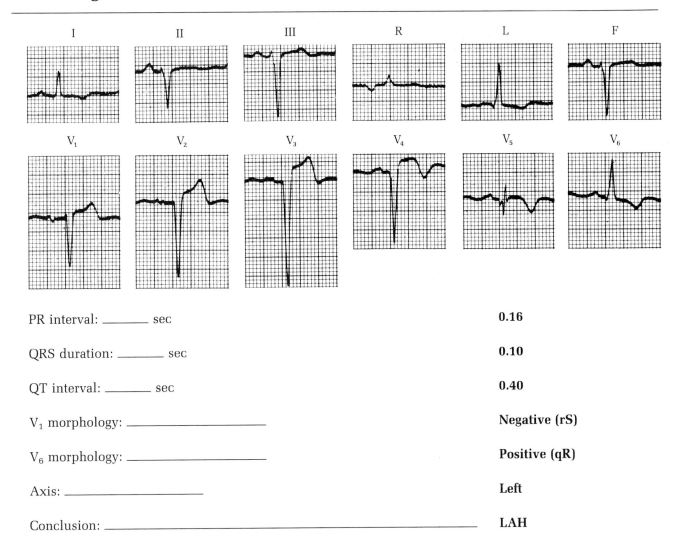

PR interval: _____ sec   **0.16**

QRS duration: _____ sec   **0.10**

QT interval: _____ sec   **0.40**

V_1 morphology: _____   **Negative (rS)**

V_6 morphology: _____   **Positive (qR)**

Axis: _____   **Left**

Conclusion: _____   **LAH**

Immediately apparent in this 12 lead ECG is the left axis deviation (LAD), as reflected by the positive complex in lead I and the negative one in lead II. This rS pattern in lead II, along with the qR pattern in lead I, is diagnostic of LAH. A glance at lead V_1 indicates that the right bundle branch is still intact. You will notice that the R wave progression in the precordial leads is lost. This may indicate an anteroseptal myocardial infarction, which is discussed in Chapter 12.

To determine the electrical axis by estimation, you would find an equiphasic deflection in one of the limb leads. Lead aV_R is not equiphasic, but it is the smallest deflection, indicating that the main current flow crosses the axis of this lead almost on a perpendicular. The axis of lead III is also perpendicular to the axis of this lead. The strong negative deflection in lead III indicates that the main current flow is toward the negative terminal of that lead, which places the electrical axis at approximately $-60°$.

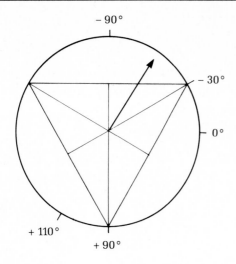

An electrical axis of $-60°$ would be perpendicular to the axis of aV_R and flowing into the negative terminal of lead III.

Tracing 7-5

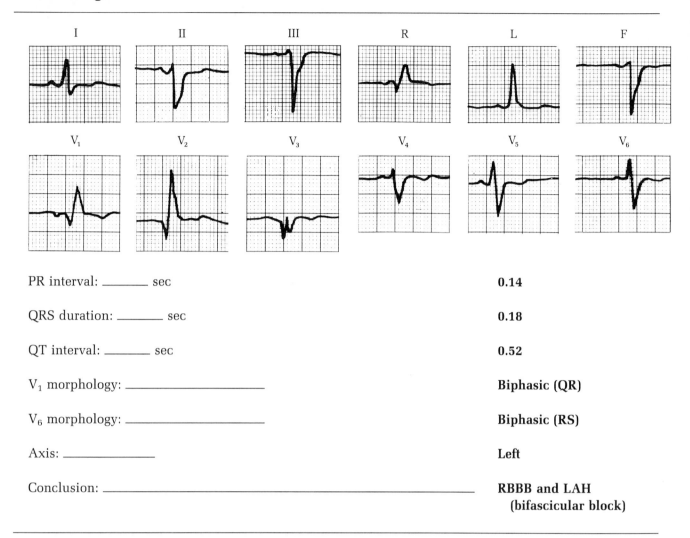

I	II	III
R	L	F
V₁	V₂	V₃
V₄	V₅	V₆

PR interval: _____ sec   **0.14**

QRS duration: _____ sec   **0.18**

QT interval: _____ sec   **0.52**

V₁ morphology: _____   **Biphasic (QR)**

V₆ morphology: _____   **Biphasic (RS)**

Axis: _____   **Left**

Conclusion: _____   **RBBB and LAH
                                                              (bifascicular block)**

The broad terminal R wave in lead V_1 indicates late activation of the right ventricle, and the positive complex in lead I and the negative one in lead II indicates LAD. The diagnosis is, then, RBBB and LAH (bifascicular block).

The electrical axis is estimated by looking at the six limb leads for an equiphasic, or nearly equiphasic, deflection. This is found in lead aV_R, where the complex is more positive than it is negative but is the closest to being isoelectric. You can therefore surmise that the main current flow is almost perpendicular to the axis of aV_R. However, you do not know whether the current goes to the left or the right. Since the axis of lead III is also perpendicular to the axis of aV_R, you have a good guide for determining the direction. Lead III is strongly negative, indicating that the current flows toward the negative terminal of this lead and thus that the axis of the heart is mainly to the left. To be more specific, you can now take into account the more positive value of aV_R and swing the axis a little more toward the lead's positive electrode, which would bring the electrical axis of the heart somewhere between $-60°$ and $-65°$.

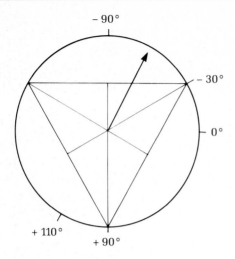

An electrical axis of $-65°$ would be almost perpendicular to the axis of aV_R and flowing toward the negative terminal of lead III.

Tracing 7-6

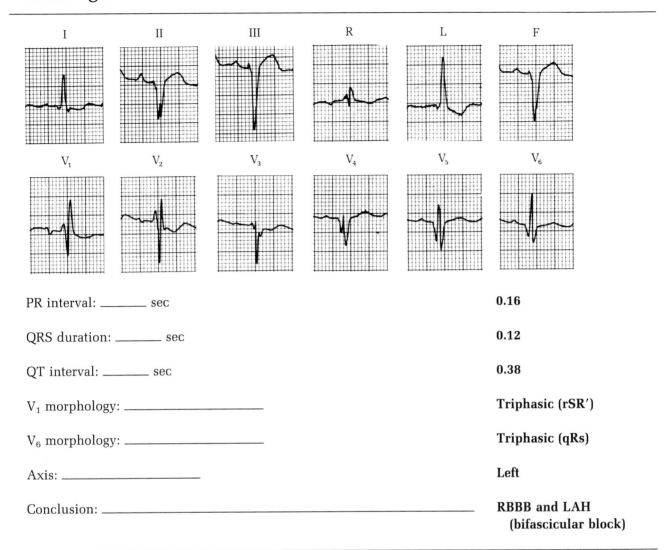

PR interval: _____ sec   **0.16**

QRS duration: _____ sec   **0.12**

QT interval: _____ sec   **0.38**

V_1 morphology: _____   **Triphasic (rSR′)**

V_6 morphology: _____   **Triphasic (qRs)**

Axis: _____   **Left**

Conclusion: _____   **RBBB and LAH**
                                                                    (bifascicular block)

In lead V_1 of this ECG it is possible to see the deflections resulting from depolarization of both the left and the right ventricles. The small initial r wave represents normal septal depolarization from left to right, or toward the positive terminal of this lead. The deep S wave reflects normal left-ventricular depolarization, and the terminal R′ wave is a telltale sign of late activation of the right ventricle (RBBB). Ordinarily, the right-ventricular force is lost in the greater force of the left ventricle when both ventricles depolarize together as they should. This delayed right-ventricular activation can also be seen in the left precordial leads and in lead I as a broad terminal S wave, reflective of a force traveling away from these positive terminals.

The electrical axis of this patient's heart is best determined from leads aV_R and III. It is almost perpendicular to the axis of aV_R and directed toward the negative terminal of III, placing the main current flow toward the left shoulder. This, combined with the qR and I and the rS in II, is diagnostic of LAH.

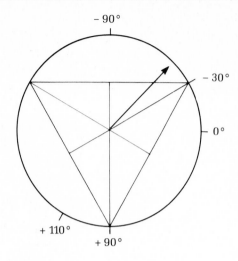

An electrical axis of $-45°$ would be perpendicular to the axis of aV_R and flowing into the positive terminal of lead III.

Tracing 7-7

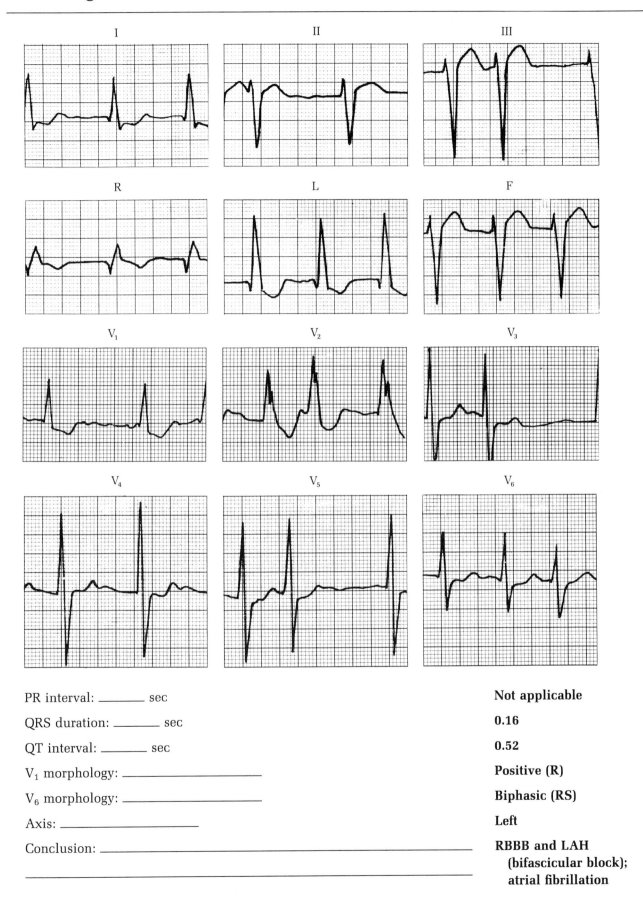

PR interval: _____ sec   **Not applicable**

QRS duration: _____ sec   **0.16**

QT interval: _____ sec   **0.52**

V₁ morphology: _____   **Positive (R)**

V₆ morphology: _____   **Biphasic (RS)**

Axis: _____   **Left**

Conclusion: _____   **RBBB and LAH
                                                (bifascicular block);
                                                atrial fibrillation**

The broad terminal R wave in lead V$_1$ is abnormal and indicates a late current flowing toward the electrode of this lead, which is a sign of late activation of the right ventricle (RBBB). Since the right bundle and the anterior division of the left bundle have a common anatomical origin and a common blood supply (anterior descending branch of the left coronary artery), you will be on the alert for a coexisting block of the left anterior fascicle. This is clearly evident in the left axis deviation. There is, then, a block of two of the fascicles of the ventricular conductive system. Ordinarily, at this point you would be concerned about the prolongation of the PR interval, indicating involvement of the only remaining fascicle. However, this patient has atrial fibrillation, and recognition of involvement of the posterior fascicle by a very slow idioventricular rhythm (trifascicular block) would probably come too late.

Estimation of the electrical axis is easily made by observing the almost equiphasic complex in aV$_R$ and the negative complex in III. These complexes indicate that the mean electrical axis is directed up toward the left shoulder, with slightly more value toward the positive pole of aV$_R$—at about −60°.

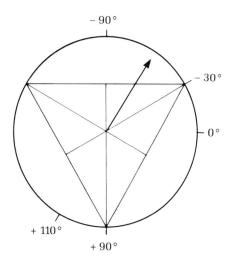

An electrical axis of −60° would be almost perpendicular to the axis of aV$_R$ and flowing more toward the negative terminal of lead III.

Tracing 7-8

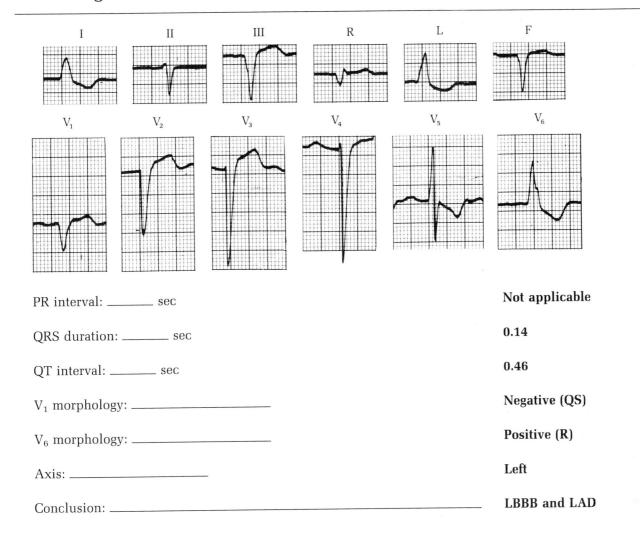

| I | II | III | R | L | F |

| V₁ | V₂ | V₃ | V₄ | V₅ | V₆ |

PR interval: _____ sec   **Not applicable**

QRS duration: _____ sec   **0.14**

QT interval: _____ sec   **0.46**

V₁ morphology: _____   **Negative (QS)**

V₆ morphology: _____   **Positive (R)**

Axis: _____   **Left**

Conclusion: _____   **LBBB and LAD**

This is LBBB with LAD. P waves are not seen because of atrial fibrillation. The axis does not always shift to the left with LBBB. Such a shift occurs in about 30% of cases.

Note the absence of Q waves in I, aV$_L$ and V$_6$, which is reflective of abnormal septal activation, expected in LBBB.

Tracing 7-9

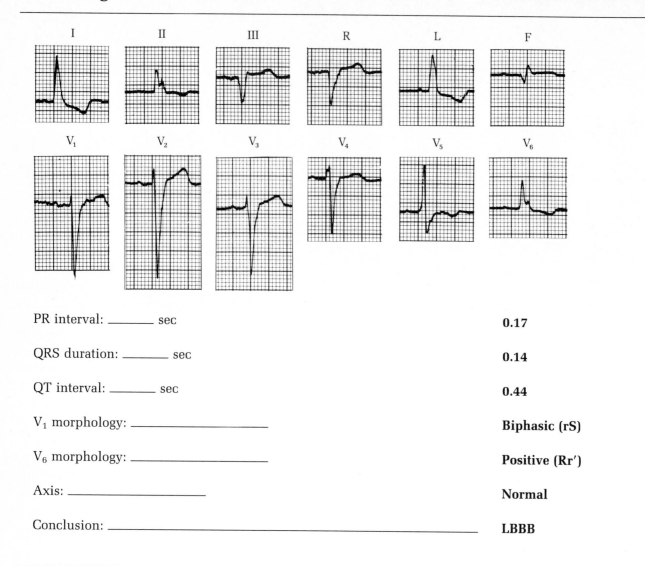

PR interval: _____ sec   **0.17**

QRS duration: _____ sec   **0.14**

QT interval: _____ sec   **0.44**

V_1 morphology: _____   **Biphasic (rS)**

V_6 morphology: _____   **Positive (Rr′)**

Axis: _____   **Normal**

Conclusion: _____   **LBBB**

Note the narrow r wave in lead V_1. This occurs about 30% of the time in LBBB and is probably reflective of initial activation of the anterior right ventricular wall. The presence of this small narrow r wave in LBBB aberration helps one to distinguish between it and right-ventricular ectopy.

Tracing 7-10

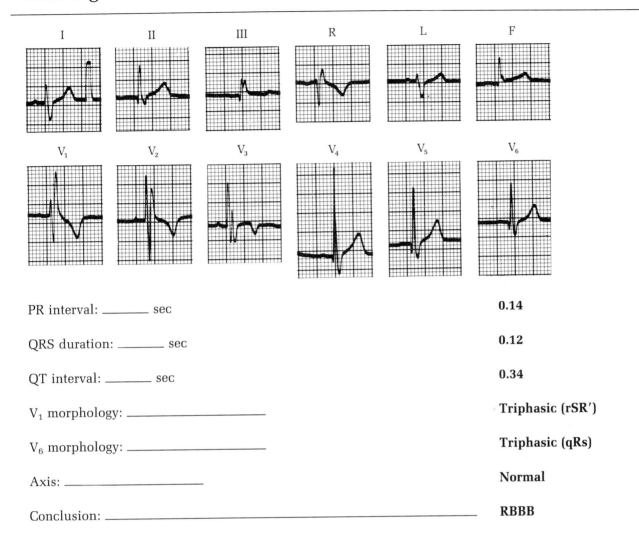

PR interval: _____ sec   **0.14**

QRS duration: _____ sec   **0.12**

QT interval: _____ sec   **0.34**

V_1 morphology: _____   **Triphasic (rSR′)**

V_6 morphology: _____   **Triphasic (qRs)**

Axis: _____   **Normal**

Conclusion: _____   **RBBB**

Watch for the development of LAD, which is reflective of LAH, by checking lead II. It is also possible that LPH could ensue. Therefore an occasional check on lead I is necessary. RAD will cause *lead I* to become almost completely negative (rS), and LAD will cause *lead II* to become almost completely negative (rS).

Tracing 7-11

II

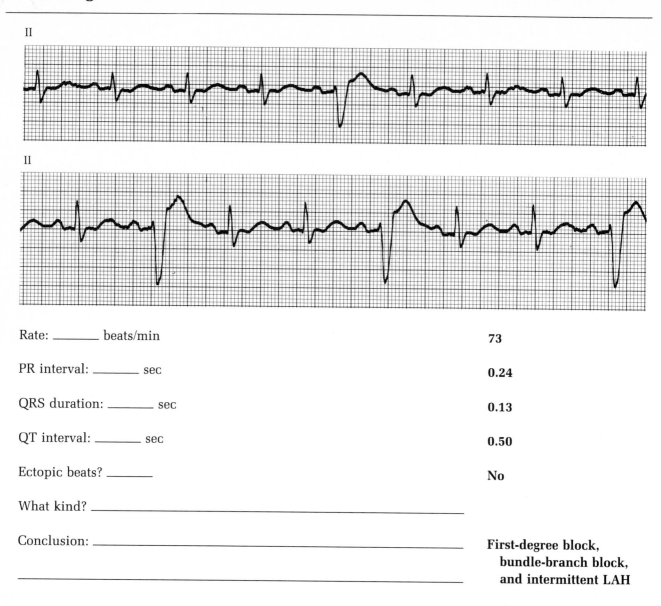

II

Rate: _____ beats/min   **73**

PR interval: _____ sec   **0.24**

QRS duration: _____ sec   **0.13**

QT interval: _____ sec   **0.50**

Ectopic beats? _____   **No**

What kind? _____

Conclusion: _____   **First-degree block,**
_____   **bundle-branch block,**
                                                     and intermittent LAH

This patient has intermittent LAH, which began with an occasional block and then occurred every third beat. There is also first-degree heart block. The 12-lead ECG on the next page is from the same patient later and indicates that the broad QRS seen in the above tracings is reflective of RBBB.

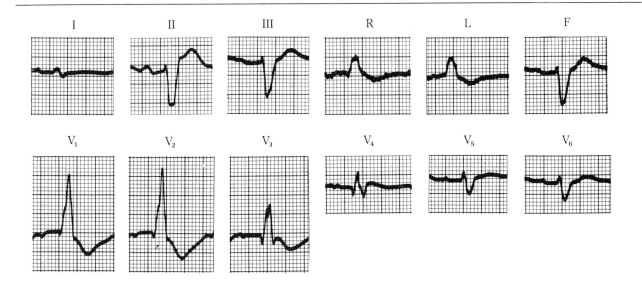

This is an example of trifascicular block—RBBB, LAH, and first-degree heart block. It is called trifascicular because two fascicles are obviously blocked, and the third (posterior division of the left bundle) probably has a partial block, reflected by the prolonged PR interval. The first-degree heart block could, of course, be in the bundle of His or above. However, with two fascicles already blocked, it is safer to consider that any further block involves the only remaining fascicle. If LPH ensues, the idioventricular rhythm may be below 30 beats/min.

Tracing 7-12

V₁

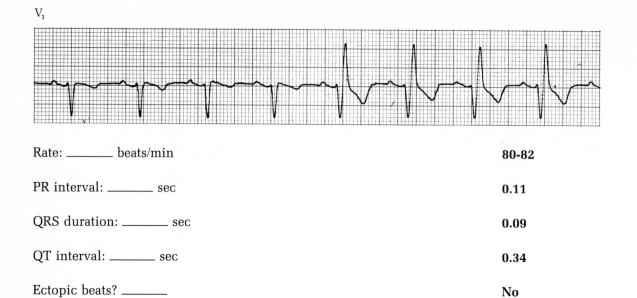

Rate: _____ beats/min   **80-82**

PR interval: _____ sec   **0.11**

QRS duration: _____ sec   **0.09**

QT interval: _____ sec   **0.34**

Ectopic beats? _____   **No**

What kind? _____

Conclusion: _____   **Rate-related RBBB**

When the cycle length shortens by only 0.04 sec, RBBB ensues. There is normal conduction at a rate of 80 beats/min, but when the heart rate increases to 82 beats/min (the "critical rate"), conduction through the right bundle branch is no longer possible.

Tracing 7-13

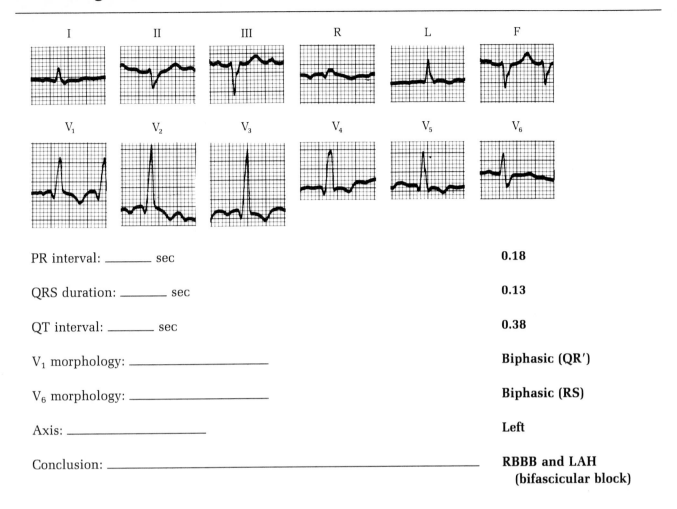

PR interval: _____ sec   **0.18**

QRS duration: _____ sec   **0.13**

QT interval: _____ sec   **0.38**

V_1 morphology: _____   **Biphasic (QR′)**

V_6 morphology: _____   **Biphasic (RS)**

Axis: _____   **Left**

Conclusion: _____   **RBBB and LAH (bifascicular block)**

Note the abnormal Q waves and the T wave inversion in the chest leads from V_1 to V_5 and the absence of normal q waves in leads I and V_6. This indicates an anteroseptal myocardial infarction and is discussed in Chapter 12.

Tracing 7-14

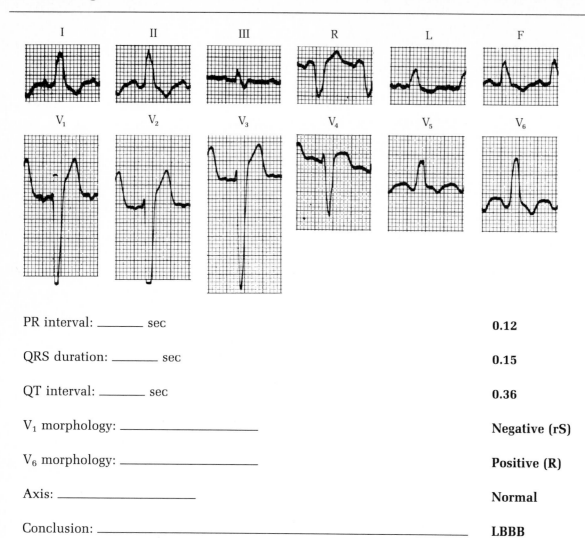

PR interval: _____ sec **0.12**

QRS duration: _____ sec **0.15**

QT interval: _____ sec **0.36**

V₁ morphology: _____ **Negative (rS)**

V₆ morphology: _____ **Positive (R)**

Axis: _____ **Normal**

Conclusion: _____ **LBBB**

Tracing 7-15

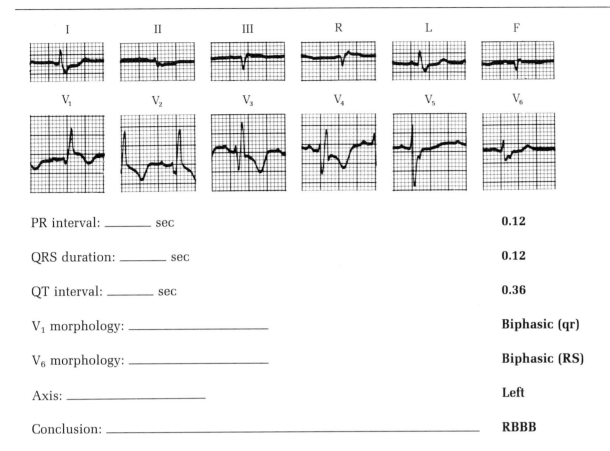

I	II	III	R	L	F

V_1	V_2	V_3	V_4	V_5	V_6

PR interval: _____ sec   **0.12**

QRS duration: _____ sec   **0.12**

QT interval: _____ sec   **0.36**

V_1 morphology: _____   **Biphasic (qr)**

V_6 morphology: _____   **Biphasic (RS)**

Axis: _____   **Left**

Conclusion: _____   **RBBB**

Tracing 7-16

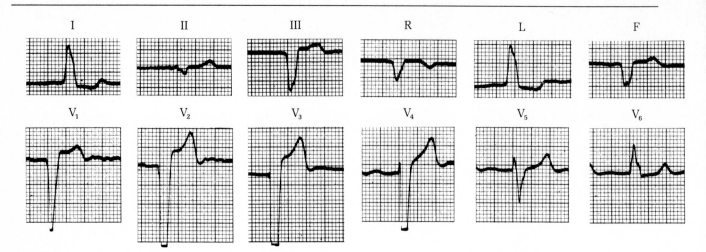

PR interval: _____ sec   **Not applicable**

QRS duration: _____ sec   **0.14**

QT interval: _____ sec   **0.48**

V_1 morphology: _____   **Negative (QS)**

V_6 morphology: _____   **Positive (R)**

Axis: _____   **Left**

Conclusion: _____   **LBBB**

Tracing 7-17

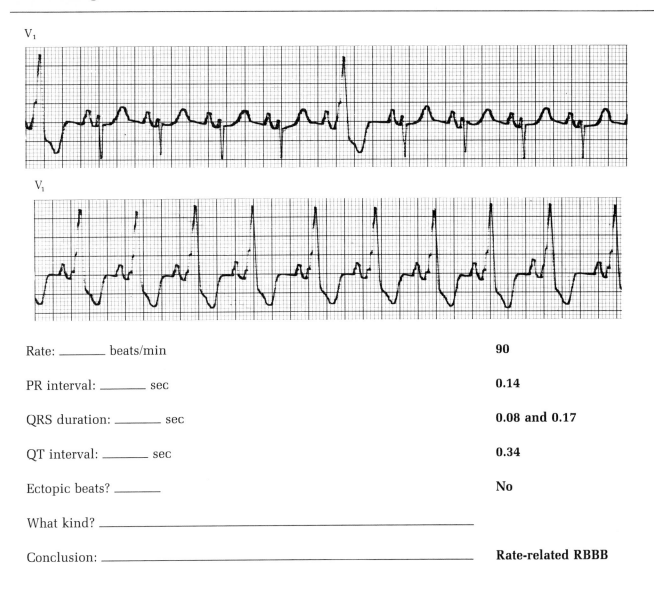

Rate: _____ beats/min **90**

PR interval: _____ sec **0.14**

QRS duration: _____ sec **0.08 and 0.17**

QT interval: _____ sec **0.34**

Ectopic beats? _____ **No**

What kind? _____

Conclusion: _____ **Rate-related RBBB**

In the top tracing, when the cycle length shortens by only 0.02 sec RBBB ensues. In the bottom tracing, there is RBBB conduction with every beat even though the heart rate has slowed from 92 beats/min to 90. The rate-dependent bundle-branch block develops at a rate faster than the rate at which it disappears, to that even though it takes a critical rate of 92 to initiate the bundle-branch block, the heart would have to slow down more than that in order to terminate it.

8

ABERRANT VENTRICULAR CONDUCTION VERSUS VENTRICULAR ECTOPY

- ☐ **RBBB aberration**
- ☐ **LBBB aberration**
- ☐ **Left-ventricular ectopy**
- ☐ **Right-ventricular ectopy**
- ☐ **Differential diagnosis**

Aberrant ventricular conduction

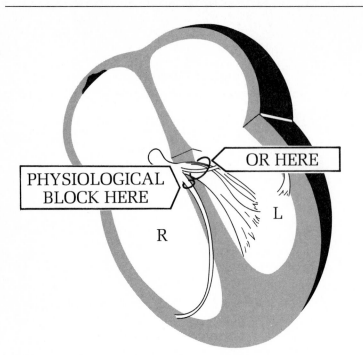

Aberrancy is the *temporary* abnormal conduction of a supraventricular complex.

PHYSIOLOGICAL BLOCK HERE

OR HERE

R

L

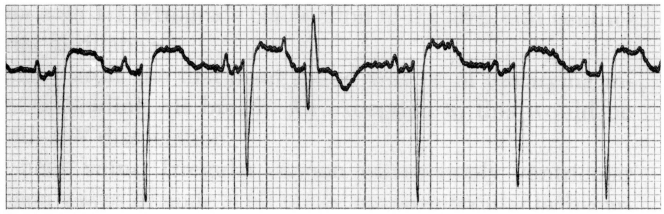

Aberrant ventricular conduction is not a _____ condition. **pathological**

Aberrant ventricular conduction occurs because of a _____ **shortening**
of the cycle length.

Aberrant ventricular conduction may be either _____ or _____ **right; left**
bundle-branch block.

ECG patterns in aberration and in ectopy

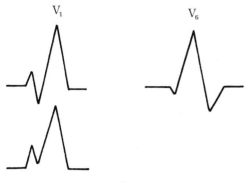

When these patterns are seen, RBBB aberration is indicated as long as the axis is not left.

RBBB aberration

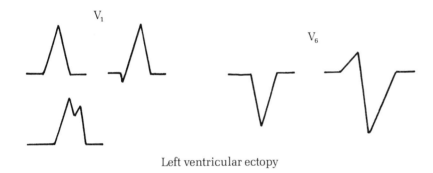

These patterns indicate left-ventricular ectopy. The axis is often left.

Left ventricular ectopy

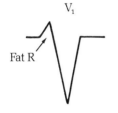

This pattern indicates right-ventricular ectopy, especially when the pattern is associated with right axis deviation.

Right ventricular ectopy

Heart rate in aberration and in ectopy

ABERRATION

> *Heart rate greater than 170; QRS 0.14 sec or less*

ECTOPY

> *Heart rate less than 170; QRS greater than 0.14 sec*

In supraventricular tachycardia the heart rate is frequently between _____ and 200 beats/min.   **170**

In ventricular tachycardia the heart rate is frequently between 130 and _____ beats/min.   **170**

In aberrancy the QRS duration is frequently _____ sec or less.   **0.14**

In ventricular tachycardia the QRS duration is frequently more than _____ sec.   **0.14**

Tracing 8-1

V₁

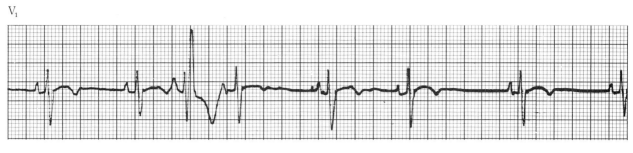

Rate: _____ beats/min	**60 (underlying)**
PR interval: _____ sec	**0.12**
QRS duration: _____ sec	**0.08**
QT interval: _____ sec	**0.37**
Ectopic beats? _____	**Yes**
What kind? _____	**Atrial**
Conclusion: _____	**PAC with RBBB aberration and a reciprocating mechanism**

The PAC before the anomalous-looking beat is easily seen. It is conducted with RBBB aberration. A reciprocating mechanism follows, consisting of a retrograde P′ and a ventricular reciprocal beat. The sinus rhythm recommences, only to be interrupted by another PAC. This time conduction is normal because the P′ wave occurs later in the cycle.

Tracing 8-2

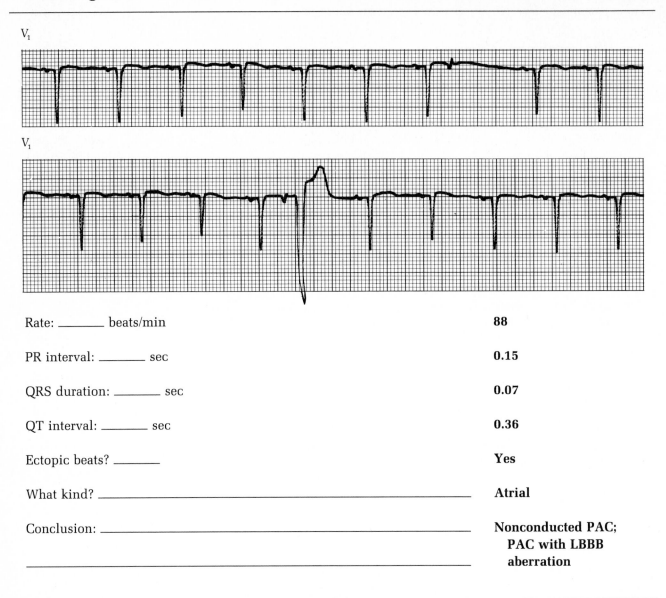

V₁

V₁

Rate: _____ beats/min	**88**
PR interval: _____ sec	**0.15**
QRS duration: _____ sec	**0.07**
QT interval: _____ sec	**0.36**
Ectopic beats? _____	**Yes**
What kind? _____	**Atrial**
Conclusion: _____	**Nonconducted PAC; PAC with LBBB aberration**

There is a nonconducted PAC in the first tracing. In the second tracing the PAC is conducted with incomplete LBBB aberration (QRS of 0.10 sec).

If the P′ wave were not so evident, the less-than-full compensatory pause would have helped to indicate atrial ectopy. Morphologically there would be no clues.

Tracing 8-3

V₁

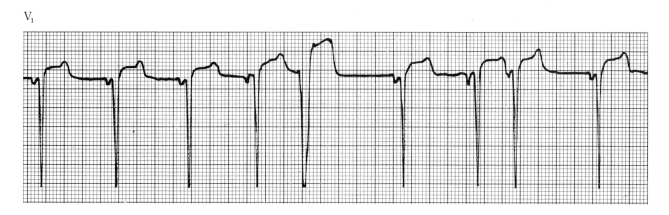

Rate: _____ beats/min

PR interval: _____ sec

QRS duration: _____ sec

QT interval: _____ sec

Ectopic beats? _____

What kind? _____

Conclusion: _____

75 (underlying)

0.09

0.06

0.37

Yes

Atrial

PACs with LBBB aberration

Two PACs in this tracing are followed by a reciprocating mechanism. The fourth P wave is premature and of a different morphology from the preceding P waves. It is followed by an atrial echo beat (in the T wave). The ventricular response (reciprocal beat) is conducted with LBBB aberration. The same sequence evolves with the next PAC (third P from the end). However, this time the reciprocal beat is conducted normally.

Tracing 8-4

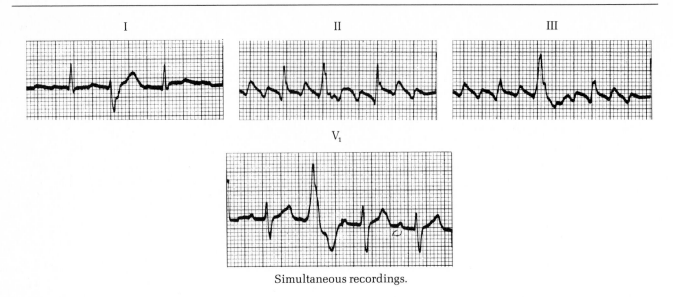

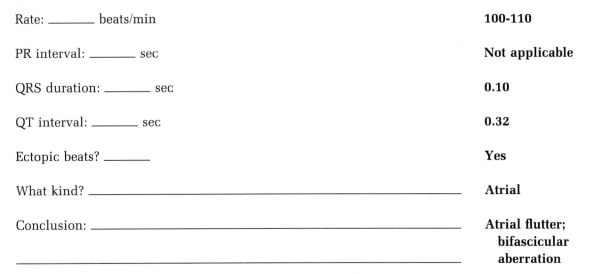

Simultaneous recordings.

Rate: _____ beats/min   **100-110**

PR interval: _____ sec   **Not applicable**

QRS duration: _____ sec   **0.10**

QT interval: _____ sec   **0.32**

Ectopic beats? _____   **Yes**

What kind? _____ **Atrial**

Conclusion: _____   **Atrial flutter;**
                                    bifascicular
_____   **aberration**

This is atrial flutter with 3:1 and 2:1 AV conduction. When conduction is 2:1, it is aberrant. The limb leads reflect LPH aberrancy, and lead V_1 reflects RBBB aberrancy. Therefore, when the conduction ratio is 2:1, the impulse is conducted only through the anterior fascicle of the left bundle. Note that the right axis deviation is picked up only in lead I. The atrial flutter waves are seen only in the inferior leads II and III. Lead I resembles atrial fibrillation, and lead V_1 looks like a sinus rhythm with first-degree heart block.

Tracing 8-5

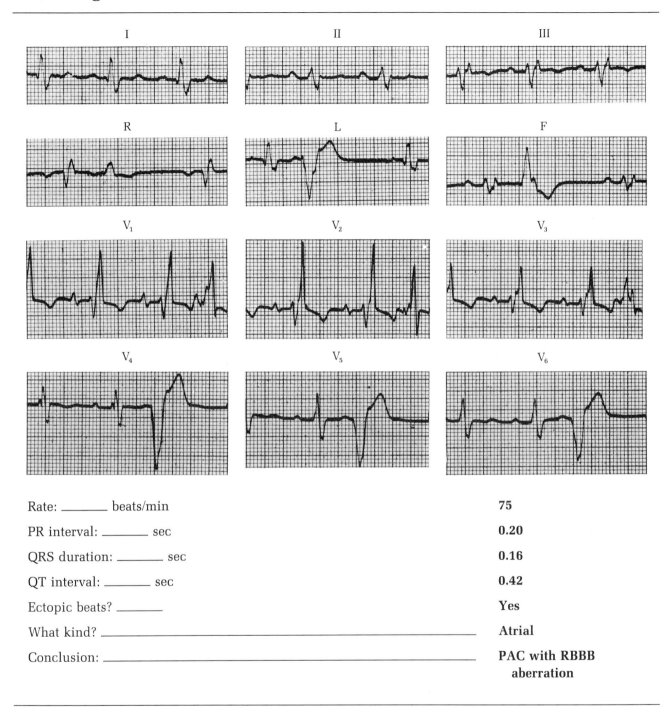

I	II	III
R	L	F
V₁	V₂	V₃
V₄	V₅	V₆

Rate: _____ beats/min   **75**

PR interval: _____ sec   **0.20**

QRS duration: _____ sec   **0.16**

QT interval: _____ sec   **0.42**

Ectopic beats? _____   **Yes**

What kind? _____   **Atrial**

Conclusion: _____   **PAC with RBBB aberration**

The broad, premature beat seen in aV_F is the result of a PAC; this conclusion is unquestionable when the beat is seen in lead V_1. In this patient the P′ wave could only be seen in the right chest leads. It is important to search not only the limb leads but also the precordial leads before you say that P waves or P′ waves are not present. Sometimes P waves are not seen in the conventional leads at all but are picked up in V_3R (same as V_3 but on right side), an S_5 (positive electrode on fifth interspace, right sternal border; negative over manubrium), or a CR connection (positive electrode on chest at V_1 position; negative at right shoulder or arm).

Tracing 8-6

V₁

V_1

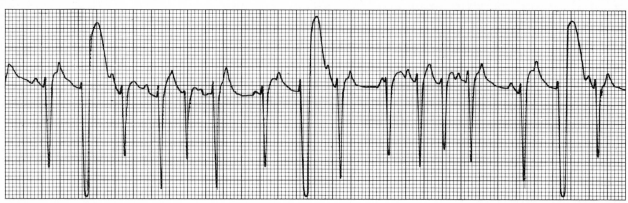

Rate: _____ beats/min	**150**
PR interval: _____ sec	**Not certain**
QRS duration: _____ sec	**0.08**
QT interval: _____ sec	**Indeterminable**
Ectopic beats? _____	**Yes**
What kind? _____	**Atrial**
Conclusion: _____ _____	**Chaotic atrial tachycardia with LBBB aberration**

The underlying arrhythmia in this tracing is chaotic atrial tachycardia (multifocal PACs). The broad complexes are supraventricular, conducted with LBBB aberration. Notice the r waves of the three complexes in question. They are narrow, reflecting initial activation of the anterior wall of the right ventricle as is sometimes seen in LBBB.

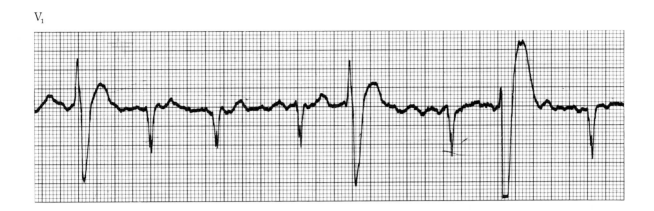

In the tracing above, atrial fibrillation is the underlying arrhythmia. The three broad complexes resemble the ones on p. 220. However, in this case the initial r waves are broad (beyond 0.03 sec). The odds now are heavily in favor of right-ventricular ectopy.

Tracing 8-7

II

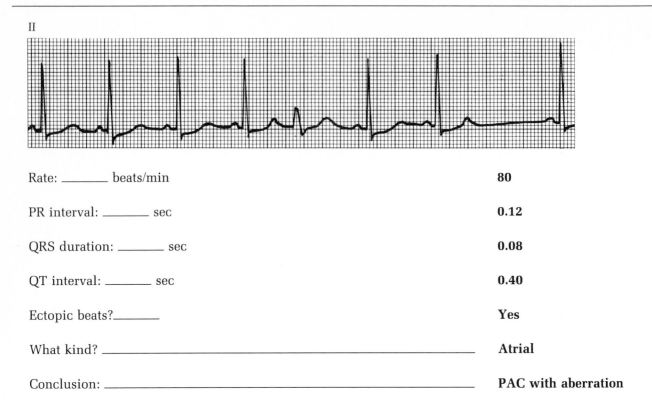

Rate: _____ beats/min   **80**

PR interval: _____ sec   **0.12**

QRS duration: _____ sec   **0.08**

QT interval: _____ sec   **0.40**

Ectopic beats?_____   **Yes**

What kind? _____   **Atrial**

Conclusion: _____   **PAC with aberration**

An abnormal complex and a pause are very apparent in this tracing. If you do not examine the tracing closely, you may decide that it shows a PVC and, later, SA block. However, even to the casual observer it should be apparent that the broad ventricular complex is not followed by a full compensatory pause, indicating premature activation of the sinus node. A comparison of the T wave morphology reveals two P′ waves in hiding. The T wave after the fourth complex is taller and more peaked than the dominant T waves. This is also seen in the T wave after the second-from-last complex. The first P′ wave is followed by aberrant ventricular conduction; the last P′ wave is not conducted at all, or perhaps it incompletely penetrates the AV junction.

The change in cycle length due to the PAC is the cause of this ventricular aberration. As the coupling interval shortens, the impulse becomes more likely to meet with incompletely repolarized tissues during its spread through the His-Purkinje system.

Tracing 8-8

II

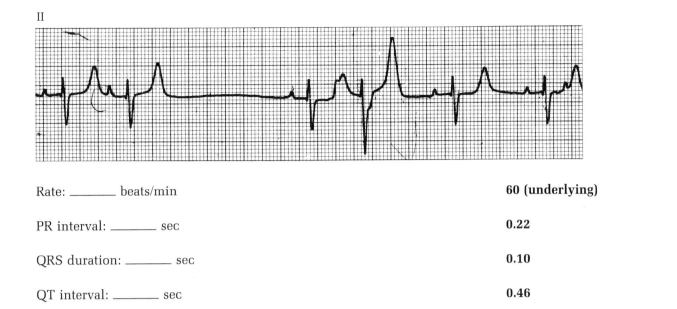

Rate: _____ beats/min

PR interval: _____ sec

QRS duration: _____ sec

QT interval: _____ sec

Ectopic beats? _____

What kind? _____

Conclusion: _____

60 (underlying)

0.22

0.10

0.46

Yes

Atrial

**Nonconducted PAC;
PAC with aberration;
first-degree block**

The second P wave in this tracing is premature and of a different morphology from the first. A nonconducted P' wave is present in the T wave preceding the pause. The next PAC (deforming the T wave of the third complex) is followed by aberrant ventricular conduction (LBBB). Two factors are causing this aberrant beat—a short coupling interval and a long preceding cycle. A long preceding cycle causes a broader action potential, which would increase the chances of a premature supraventricular impulse's meeting with tissues that are still repolarizing.

The third P' wave in this tracing is so premature that it is not conducted at all (not shown). This PAC occurs just before the last T wave.

Tracing 8-9

II

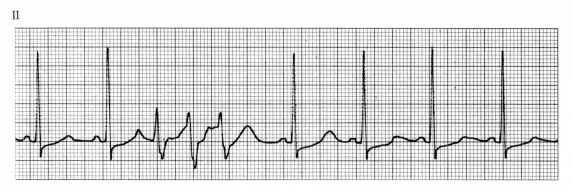

Rate: _____ beats/min   **78 (underlying)**

PR interval: _____ sec   **0.15**

QRS duration: _____ sec   **0.08**

QT interval: _____ sec   **0.52**

Ectopic beats? _____   **Yes**

What kind? _____   **Atrial**

Conclusion: _____   **PSVT with aberration**

The peaked T wave in front of the burst of tachycardia is a telltale sign of a hidden P′ wave. This P′ is followed by three aberrantly conducted beats, probably an AV nodal reciprocating mechanism.

Tracing 8-10

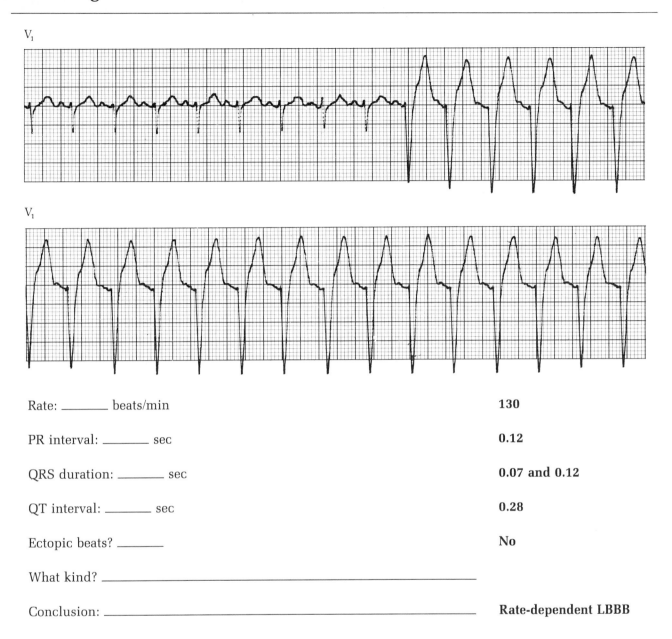

Rate: _____ beats/min   **130**

PR interval: _____ sec   **0.12**

QRS duration: _____ sec   **0.07 and 0.12**

QT interval: _____ sec   **0.28**

Ectopic beats? _____   **No**

What kind? _____

Conclusion: _____   **Rate-dependent LBBB**

In this tracing we see the onset of rate-related LBBB, which occurs when the sinus rate increases slightly. The bottom tracing could easily be mistaken for ventricular tachycardia. However, with the onset in view, there is no question that this is a supraventricular tachycardia.

Tracing 8-11

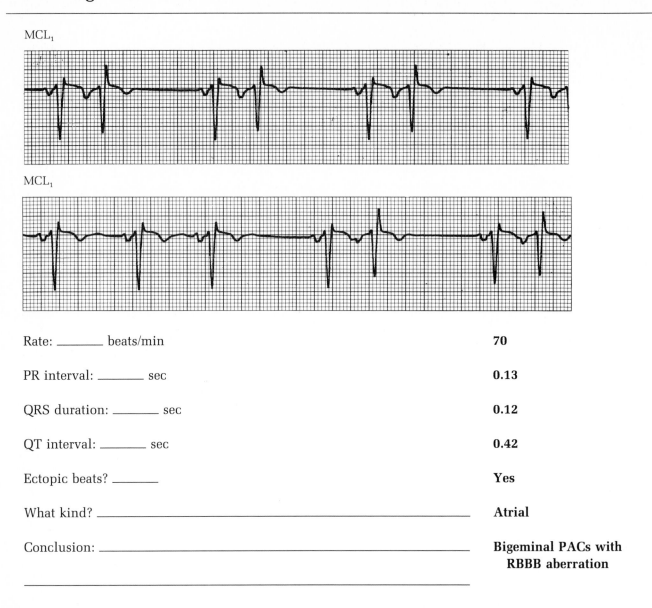

MCL₁

MCL₁

Rate: _____ beats/min   **70**

PR interval: _____ sec   **0.13**

QRS duration: _____ sec   **0.12**

QT interval: _____ sec   **0.42**

Ectopic beats? _____   **Yes**

What kind? _____   **Atrial**

Conclusion: _____   **Bigeminal PACs with
                                                                           RBBB aberration**

_____

   The genesis of the bigeminal rhythm in the first tracing becomes more
readily apparent when you look at the second tracing (from the same patient), in which the first four complexes are normal sinus in origin. These
are followed by bigeminal PACs, all of which are conducted with more
RBBB than is already present in the dominant rhythm.

Tracing 8-12

II

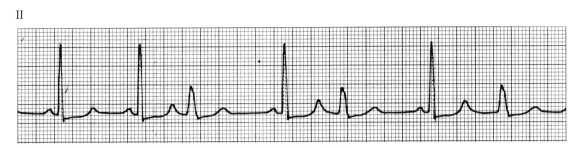

Rate: _____ beats/min   **75 (underlying)**

PR interval: _____ sec   **0.16**

QRS duration: _____ sec   **0.07**

QT interval: _____ sec   **0.42**

Ectopic beats? _____   **Yes**

What kind? _____   **Atrial**

Conclusion: _____   **Bigeminal PACs with**
                                                             aberration

_____

Here again, as in the Tracing 8-11, the bigeminal rhythm is due to PACs conducted aberrantly through the ventricles. The first two complexes are normally conducted sinus beats; afterward a change in the shape of the T wave is noted, indicative of a hidden P′ wave. The impulse is conducted aberrantly because of the short coupling interval along with the abrupt change in cycle length.

Tracing 8-13

II

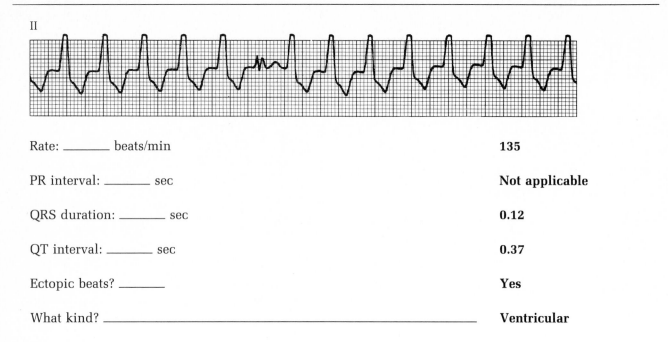

Rate: _____ beats/min   **135**

PR interval: _____ sec   **Not applicable**

QRS duration: _____ sec   **0.12**

QT interval: _____ sec   **0.37**

Ectopic beats? _____   **Yes**

What kind? _____   **Ventricular**

Conclusion: _____   **Ventricular tachycardia**

There is a (ventricular fusion beat) present in this tracing, as reflected in the narrower complex of lesser amplitude. This could indicate one of two possibilities. The first is that during ventricular tachycardia, a sinus impulse partially captured the ventricles; that is, a sinus impulse has found the AV junction nonrefractory and has descended and fused with the ectopic activity. The second possibility is that this tracing represents a supraventricular tachycardia and that a ventricular ectopic beat has discharged at the same time, causing a fusion of the supraventricular pacemaker vector and the ventricular ectopic vector. Thus the arrhythmia may be either ventricular or supraventricular with aberration. Unless there are morphological clues in lead V_1 or V_6 strongly favoring aberration, this arrhythmia should be treated aggressively as a ventricular tachycardia. Aberrancy should never be diagnosed without proof.

Tracing 8-14

V_1

V_2

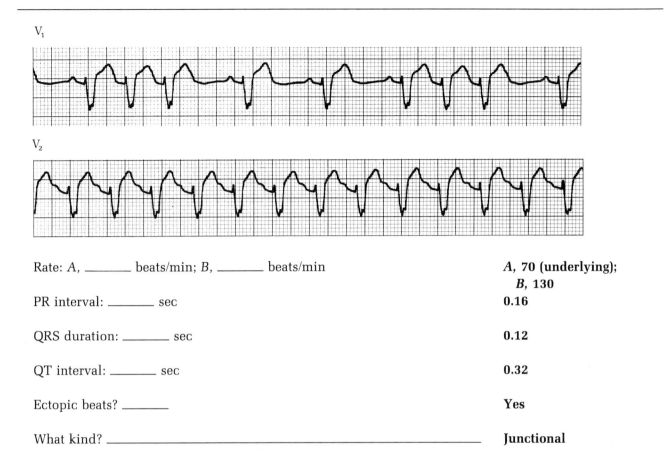

Rate: A, _____ beats/min; B, _____ beats/min   **A, 70 (underlying);**
    B, 130

PR interval: _____ sec   **0.16**

QRS duration: _____ sec   **0.12**

QT interval: _____ sec   **0.32**

Ectopic beats? _____   **Yes**

What kind? _____   **Junctional**

Conclusion: _____   **SVT**

A look at the isolated extrasystoles leaves no doubt as to the origin of this tachycardia. The dominant rhythm in the first tracing is a sinus rhythm with a broad QRS. Premature junctional beats are present, which are paired and conducted with the same broad pattern as the sinus-conducted beats. Identical complexes are seen in the tachycardia, which resemble those of ventricular tachycardia because of their broad morphology but which are those of supraventricular tachycardia (SVT).

Tracing 8-15

V₁

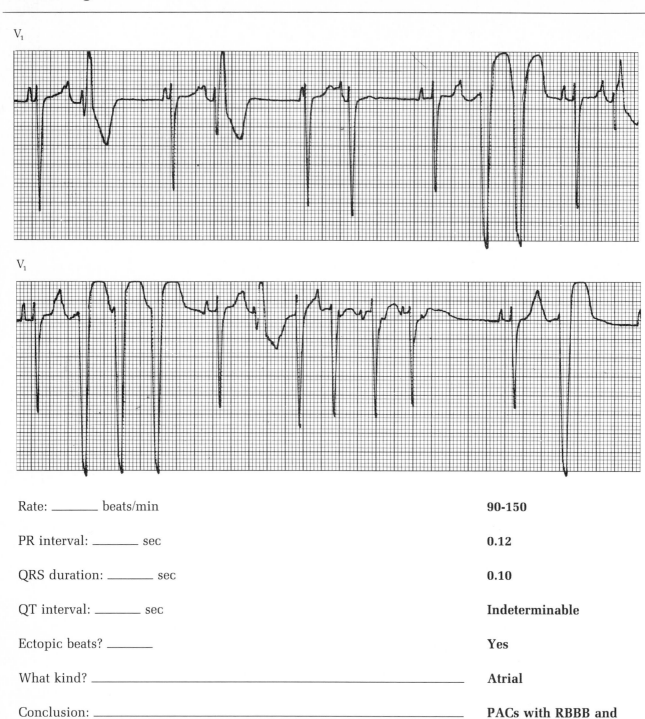

V₁

Rate: _____ beats/min   **90-150**

PR interval: _____ sec   **0.12**

QRS duration: _____ sec   **0.10**

QT interval: _____ sec   **Indeterminable**

Ectopic beats? _____   **Yes**

What kind? _____   **Atrial**

Conclusion: _____   **PACs with RBBB and**
                                                       LBBB aberration

The PACs are very evident in this tracing, distorting the T waves. They are conducted with both RBBB and LBBB aberration.

In the bottom tracing the first beat is sinus conducted. There is a P' wave in the T wave, which initiates a burst of supraventricular tachycardia. The first three complexes of the tachycardia are conducted with LBBB aberration. The fourth beat is conducted normally and then with RBBB aberration. The remainder of the tachycardia is conducted normally and with incomplete LBBB aberration.

Tracing 8-16

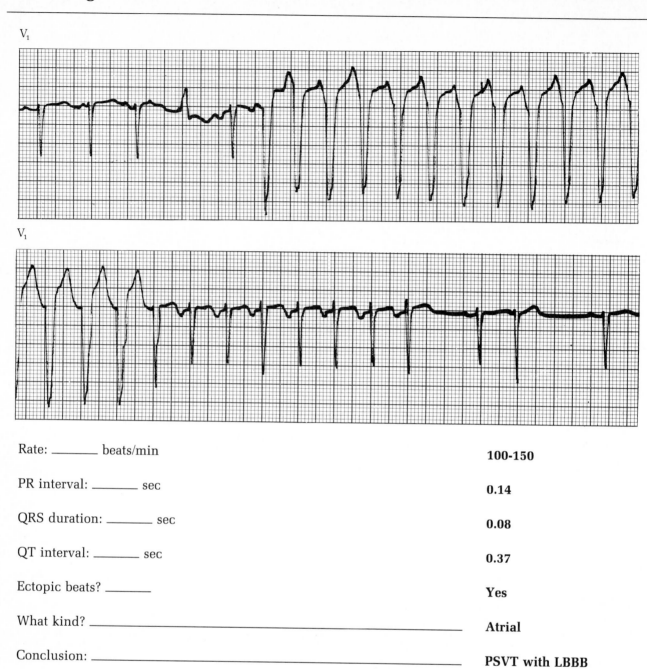

V$_1$

V$_1$

Rate: _____ beats/min

PR interval: _____ sec

QRS duration: _____ sec

QT interval: _____ sec

Ectopic beats? _____

What kind? _____

Conclusion: _____

100-150

0.14

0.08

0.37

Yes

Atrial

**PSVT with LBBB
aberration**

This is a paroxysmal supraventricular tachycardia with LBBB aberration. The first three beats are sinus. There is a P′ wave in the third T,
followed by a supraventricular beat of RBBB configuration. This begins a
rapid AV nodal reentry mechanism, which is clearly seen as it ends in
normal conduction in the second tracing.

Tracing 8-17

I

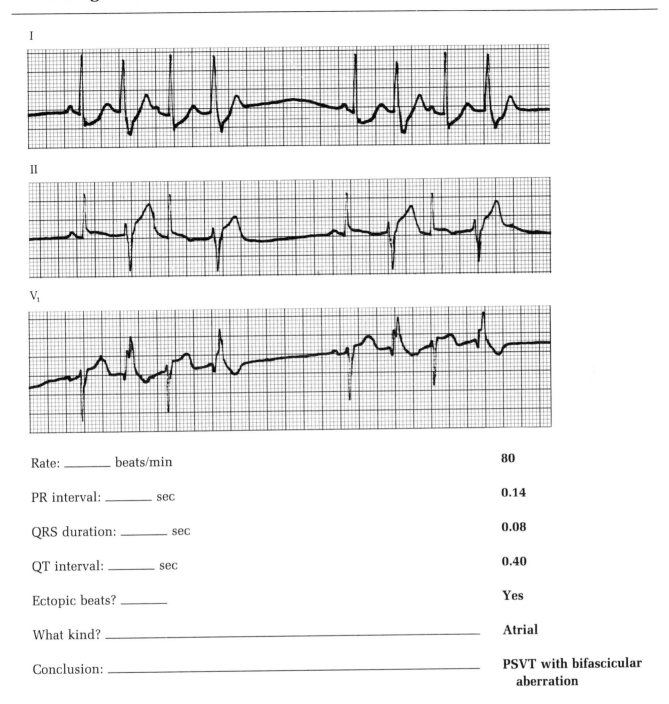

II

V₁

Rate: _____ beats/min	**80**
PR interval: _____ sec	**0.14**
QRS duration: _____ sec	**0.08**
QT interval: _____ sec	**0.40**
Ectopic beats? _____	**Yes**
What kind? _____	**Atrial**
Conclusion: _____	**PSVT with bifascicular aberration**

This patient had bursts of supraventricular tachycardia, which always terminated after 3 beats. In lead I every other beat is broadened by an s wave. This is the typical morphology of RBBB in leads I and V_6. Lead II indicates that the broad beats have LAD, reflective of LAH. In lead V_1 the broad beats in question are primarily positive. P′ waves can be seen in all three leads. They are conducted with bifascicular block (LAH and RBBB aberration).

Tracing 8-18

V₁

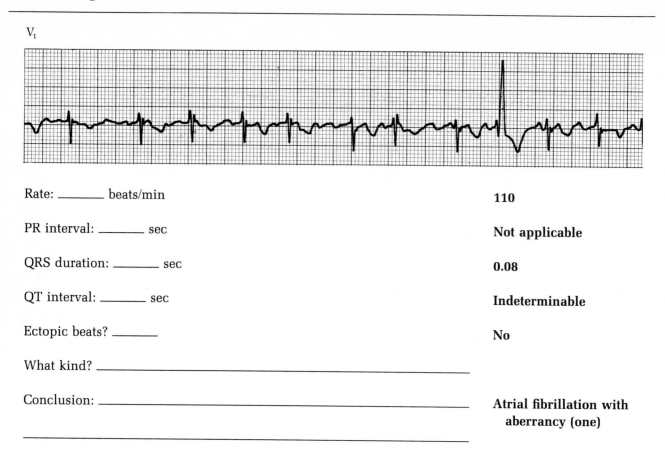

Rate: _____ beats/min

110

PR interval: _____ sec

Not applicable

QRS duration: _____ sec

0.08

QT interval: _____ sec

Indeterminable

Ectopic beats? _____

No

What kind? _____

Conclusion: _____

Atrial fibrillation with aberrancy (one)

_____

This is atrial fibrillation with one aberrantly conducted beat (RBBB). The broad complex toward the end of the tracing has the classical RBBB pattern, as seen in lead V₁. That is, initial forces are normal, and terminal forces are late and to the right.

9

ACCESSORY PATHWAYS

- ☐ **Classical ECG in Wolff-Parkinson-White syndrome**
- ☐ **AV reentry tachycardia**
- ☐ **Normal ECG with an accessory pathway**
- ☐ **WPW syndrome and atrial fibrillation**

Wolff-Parkinson-White syndrome

Short PR; broad QRS; delta wave; tendency to PSVT.

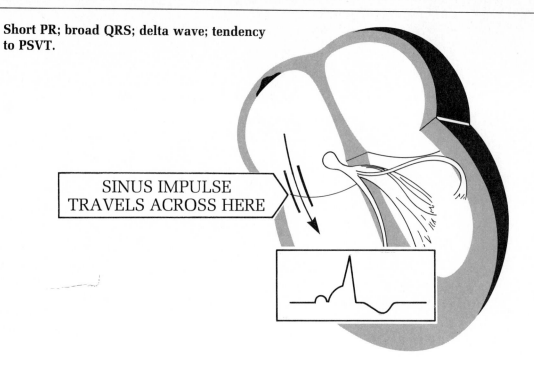

SINUS IMPULSE
TRAVELS ACROSS HERE

In Wolff-Parkinson-White (WPW) syndrome the PR is _____ because the sinus impulse enters the ventricles via an accessory pathway.

short

Conduction across the accessory pathway is faster than through the _____ node.

AV

The QRS is _____ because ventricular activation is abnormal.

broad

The initial slurring of the QRS is called a _____ wave.

delta

AV reentry tachycardia

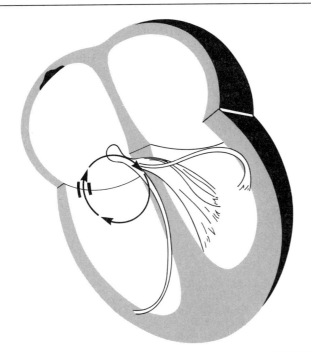

In WPW syndrome there is a tendency to PSVT.

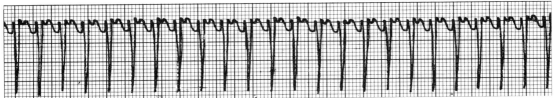

The tendency to PSVT is due to the fact that there are _____ anatomically distinct electrical pathways connecting the atria and the ventricles.

two

The PSVT may be initiated by a PAC, a PVC, or a premature junctional beat. The usual route of the reentry loop is _____ the AV node and _____ the accessory pathway.

down

up

It may be possible to interrupt this tachycardia with a vagal maneuver, which would _____ the refractory period of the AV node and interrupt the reentry loop.

lengthen

Because the usual pathway of the reentry loop is down the AV node and up the accessory pathway, the QRS complexes during the tachycardia will be of _____ configuration unless they are aberrantly conducted.

normal

NOTE: *Aberrant ventricular conduction during the AV tachycardia of WPW syndrome occurs about 70% of the time.*

An accessory pathway with normal PR, QRS, and T

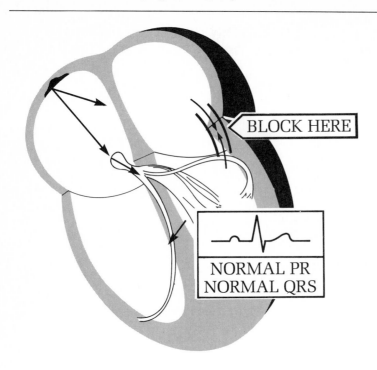

BLOCK HERE

NORMAL PR
NORMAL QRS

If the sinus impulse activates the ventricles normally before it can reach the ventricles via the accessory pathway, *the ECG will be normal.* The patient would still have the tendency to develop an AV reentry tachycardia.

If a patient has a tendency to PSVT, one should suspect and rule out _____ syndrome even if the ECG is normal.

WPW

The ECG may be normal because the sinus impulse takes longer to reach the ventricles via the _____ pathway than it does via the _____ pathway.

accessory
normal

WPW syndrome and atrial fibrillation

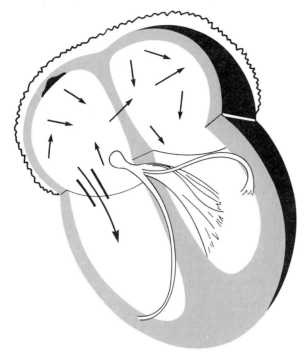

If atrial fibrillation develops, heart rates could exceed 250 beats/min.

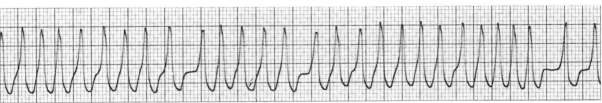

During atrial fibrillation the impulses enter the ventricles via the _____ pathway.   **accessory**

Therefore, the QRS complexes will be _____ and the rhythm will be _____.   **broad**
    irregular

The ventricular rate may be in excess of 220 beats/min because the accessory pathway does not offer the same protection as the _____ _____.   **AV node**

This is not a reentry circuit, and the AV node is not a factor; therefore a _____ maneuver will not help.   **vagal**

The ECG signs of atrial fibrillation with conduction over an accessory pathway are:
  Heart rate: _____ beats/min   **greater than 220**
  Rhythm: _____   **irregular**
  QRS: _____   **broad**

The ECG in atrial fibrillation with conduction over an accessory pathway differs from that of ventricular tachycardia, in which the rhythm is usually _____ and the rate not over _____ beats/min.   **regular; 170**

Tracing 9-1

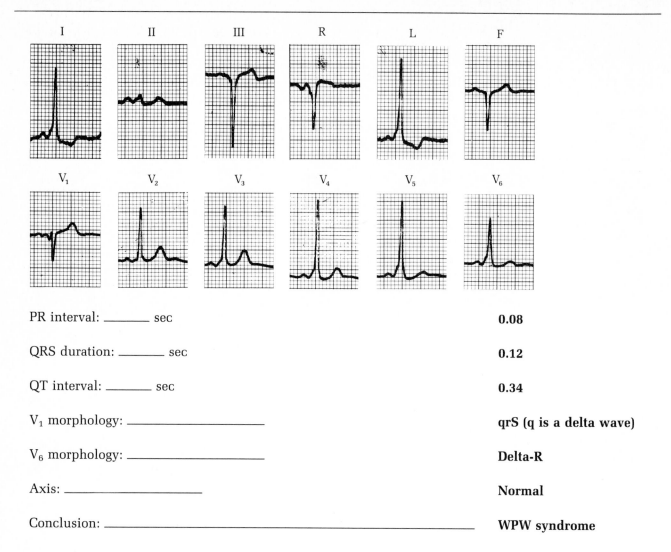

PR interval: _____ sec   **0.08**

QRS duration: _____ sec   **0.12**

QT interval: _____ sec   **0.34**

V_1 morphology: _____   **qrS (q is a delta wave)**

V_6 morphology: _____   **Delta-R**

Axis: _____   **Normal**

Conclusion: _____   **WPW syndrome**

This is Wolff-Parkinson-White (WPW) syndrome, type B (negative delta wave in V_1). It must be differentiated from inferior-wall myocardial infarction because of the pathological Q waves that sometimes appear in the inferior leads. These Q waves are really the result of the slurred initial component of the QRS complex, known as a delta wave.

Delta waves can be seen in this ECG in all leads. Other signs of Wolff-Parkinson-White syndrome are the short PR interval and the long QRS duration.

Tracing 9-2

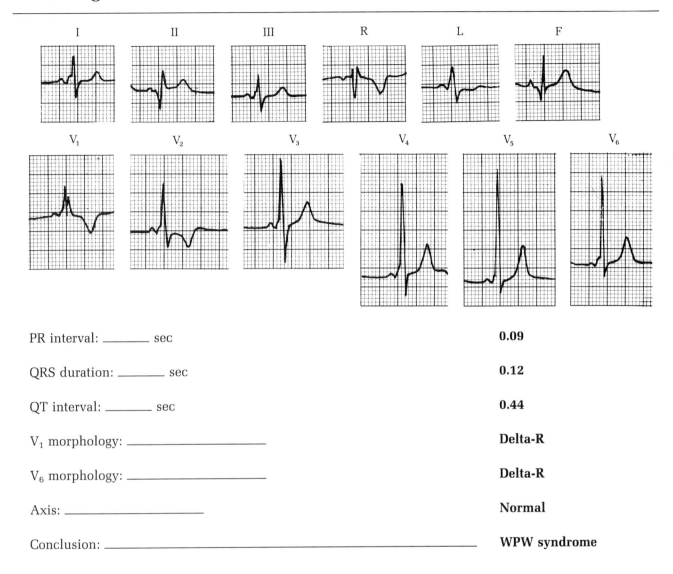

PR interval: _____ sec   **0.09**

QRS duration: _____ sec   **0.12**

QT interval: _____ sec   **0.44**

V$_1$ morphology: _____   **Delta-R**

V$_6$ morphology: _____   **Delta-R**

Axis: _____   **Normal**

Conclusion: _____   **WPW syndrome**

Here again is a Wolff-Parkinson-White syndrome. The positive QRS in lead V$_1$ indicates a type A. The presence of all of the classical signs of preexcitation (short PR, long QRS, and delta waves) would differentiate this tracing from inferior-wall myocardial infarction. The differentiation is necessary because of the abnormal Q waves (delta forces) in leads II and aV$_F$.

Tracing 9-3

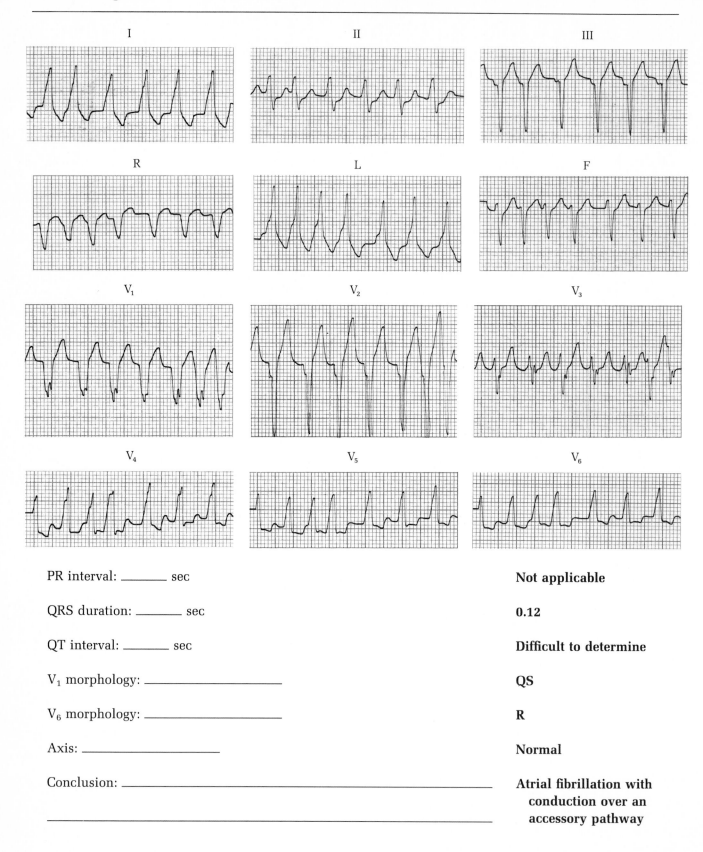

PR interval: _____ sec

QRS duration: _____ sec

QT interval: _____ sec

V₁ morphology: _____

V₆ morphology: _____

Axis: _____

Conclusion: _____

_____

Not applicable

0.12

Difficult to determine

QS

R

Normal

Atrial fibrillation with conduction over an accessory pathway

The diagnostic clues are broad QRS, irregular rhythm, and rate in excess of 220 beats/min. The atria are fibrillating; therefore the ventricular response is irregular. AV conduction is across an accessory pathway, causing a broad QRS complex. The rate is rapid because the ventricles do not have the protection of the AV node.

The ECG following cardioversion can be seen below. Note the classical features of WPW syndrome. However, remember that a normal 12-lead ECG would not have ruled out conduction over an accessory pathway during the atrial fibrillation (see p. 238).

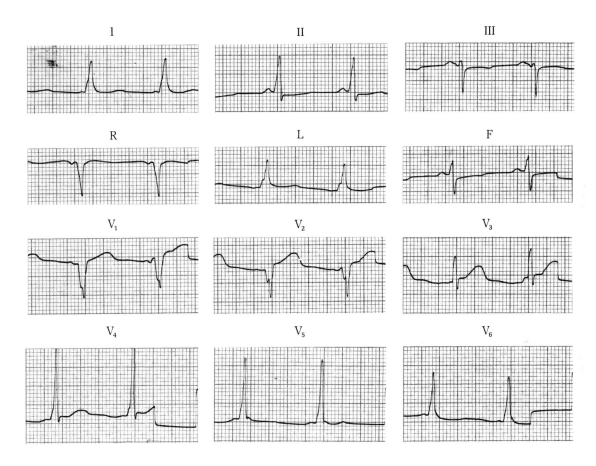

10

FUSION COMPLEXES

☐ **Mechanism of fusion**
☐ **Recognition of fusion**

Ventricular fusion

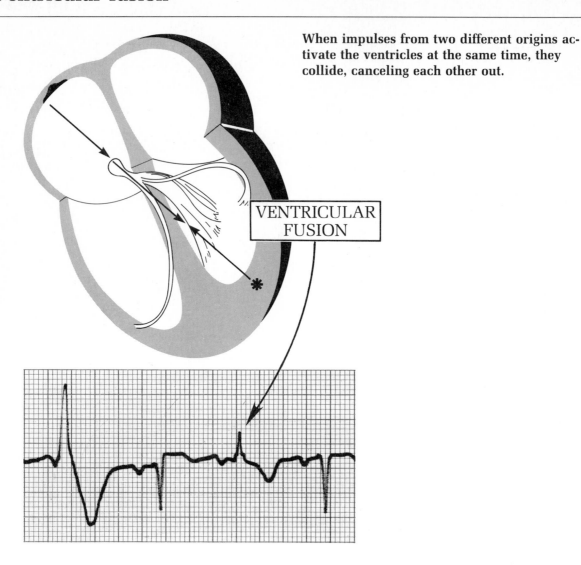

When impulses from two different origins activate the ventricles at the same time, they collide, canceling each other out.

VENTRICULAR FUSION

A ventricular fusion beat is the result of a supraventricular impulse and a _____ impulse activating the ventricles at the same time.   **ventricular**

A fusion beat is part _____ and part normal.   **ectopic**

A fusion beat may or may not be premature. If it is premature, it is generally premature by no more than 0.06 sec or so. If it is more premature than this, it activates the whole ventricle and blocks the descending _____ impulse.   **sinus**

When a fusion beat is not premature, the ectopic focus has fired at the same time or immediately _____ the supraventricular impulse has entered the ventricles.   **after**

Tracing 10-1

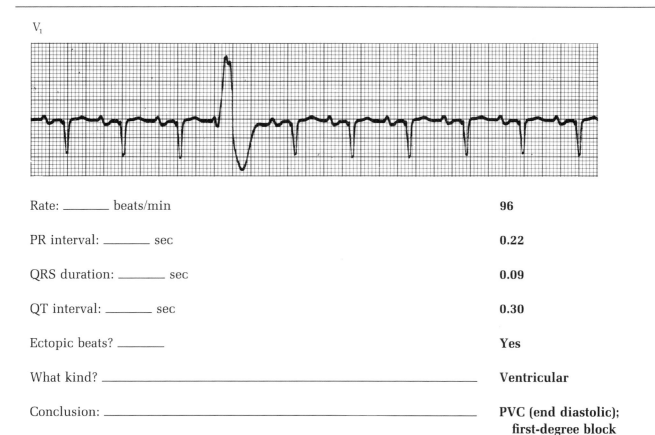

V₁

Rate: _____ beats/min	**96**
PR interval: _____ sec	**0.22**
QRS duration: _____ sec	**0.09**
QT interval: _____ sec	**0.30**
Ectopic beats? _____	**Yes**
What kind? _____	**Ventricular**
Conclusion: _____	**PVC (end diastolic); first-degree block**

The type of PVC (end diastolic) seen in this tracing probably causes more diagnostic confusion than any other. This is mainly because it is preceded by a P wave and may, therefore, as in the tracing below from the same patient, be a fusion beat.

V₁

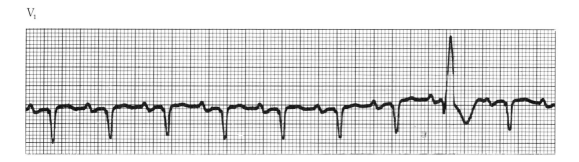

The same end-diastolic PVC is present in this tracing. However, this time it is a little later in the cycle and is now a fusion beat. If you had not noticed the change in PR intervals, you might have mistaken this for intermittent bundle-branch block.

Tracing 10-2

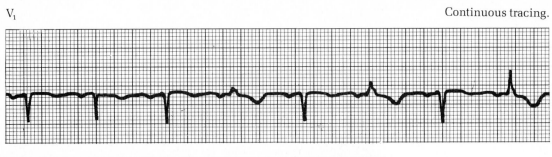

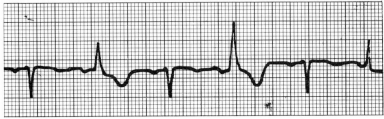

Rate: _____ beats/min   **78**

PR interval: _____ sec   **0.15**

QRS duration: _____ sec   **0.09**

QT interval: _____ sec   **0.40**

Ectopic beats? _____   **Yes**

What kind? _____   **Ventricular**

Conclusion: _____   **Bigeminal end-diastolic PVCs**

_____

The end-diastolic PVCs in this tracing occur in a bigeminal pattern, and almost all are fusion beats. Begin analyzing this arrhythmia by walking out the P waves. This is important because the sinus rhythm is perceived to be irregular when there are anomalous-looking beats following P waves. In this case it is absolutely regular. Go on to establish what is happening with AV conduction. You will notice that the PR shortens by 0.02 sec with the broad beats. This is because a ventricular ectopic beat has fired before the sinus-conducted impulse reached the ventricles. Because the PVC is only slightly premature, it does not capture all of the ventricular myocardium. The sinus-conducted impulse will also partially conduct, causing a collision of opposing electrical currents (a fusion beat). Notice that all of the fusion beats are different from each other. This is because the ectopic focus and the sinus-conducted impulse never capture exactly the same amount of myocardium. Each beat is slightly different.

Notice the first fusion beat in the second complex, which is narrower than the flanking ones. Now skip across the tracing, looking at every other beat until finally in the second strip the tallest complex looks almost totally ectopic, although it is probably still a fusion beat.

Of all the arrhythmias, bigeminal end-diastolic PVCs present one of the most confusing pictures. You should approach the tracing step by step in a logical manner until you have determined how the sinus node is functioning and whether AV conduction and ventricular conduction are occurring normally. You will meet with this arrhythmia again.

Tracing 10-3

Continuous tracing.

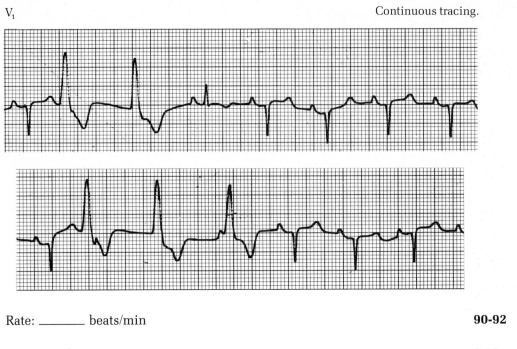

Rate: _____ beats/min   **90-92**

PR interval: _____ sec   **0.16**

QRS duration: _____ sec   **0.06**

QT interval: _____ sec   **0.34**

Ectopic beats? _____   **Yes**

What kind? _____   **Ventricular**

Conclusion: _____   **Accelerated
                                                                 idioventricular
_____   rhythm**

Here is another kind of a PVC that can cause fusion beats. It is the accelerated idioventricular rhythm (AIVR). This term implies that there is an area of enhanced automaticity within the ventricles that sometimes takes over as pacemaker at a rate that is less than 100 beats/min but that exceeds its own inherent one. This arrhythmia can manifest itself in different ways. Sometimes it appears to be more active and will begin with a very premature ventricular ectopic beat. At other times it will begin more passively, in response to a pause in the sinus rhythm. However, it is not truly an escape mechanism, because its rate is too fast.

In this tracing there is an underlying sinus rate of 90 beats/min and an ectopic ventricular focus with an accelerated rate of 75 beats/min. In the first tracing there are three PVCs from the accelerated ventricular focus; one of them is a fusion beat and follows as P wave (it is the forth complex). In the second tracing (continuous with the first) three PVCs are again seen. The coupling interval for the first PVC of each group is the same. This may indicate that the arrhythmia is initiated by a reentry mechanism. Usually, an AIVR begins as an end-diastolic PVC, rather than so prematurely, as in this example, which raises the possibility of parasystole (see p. 260).

Tracing 10-4

V₁

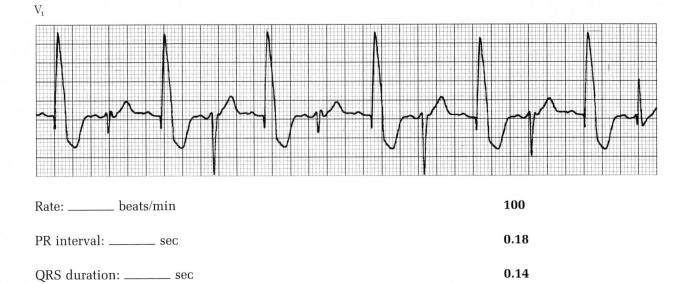

Rate: _____ beats/min   **100**

PR interval: _____ sec   **0.18**

QRS duration: _____ sec   **0.14**

QT interval: _____ sec   **0.36**

Ectopic beats? _____   **Yes**

What kind? _____   **Ventricular**

Conclusion: _____   **PVCs (end-diastolic)**

Here again is a rhythm strip reflecting bigeminal end-diastolic PVCs, which are fusion beats. At first you might think that the broad upright complexes are the ventricular ectopics. These are the sinus-conducted beats with an abnormally prolonged QRS. By walking out the P waves you will establish that the sinus rhythm is indeed regular even though it is perceived to be irregular. When you measure the PR intervals, you will find that they are absolutely fixed before the broad upright beats but that they change before the narrower beats of varying morphology. These narrow beats are fusion beats caused by frequent ventricular ectopy and should be treated as such. Also, the ventricular focus is on the same side as the bundle-branch block (and thus normalizes the QRS complex).

Tracing 10-5

II

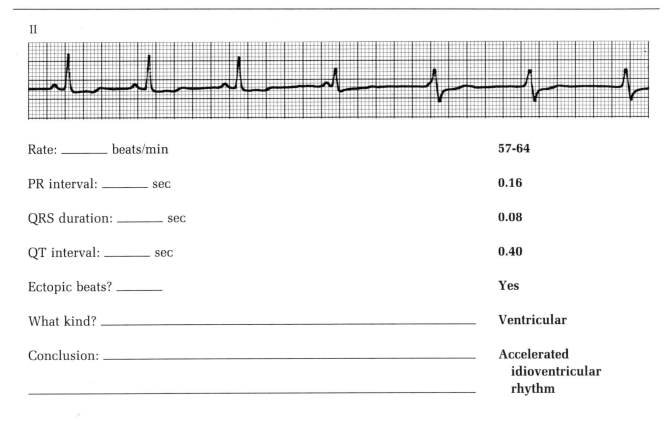

Rate: _____ beats/min	**57-64**
PR interval: _____ sec	**0.16**
QRS duration: _____ sec	**0.08**
QT interval: _____ sec	**0.40**
Ectopic beats? _____	**Yes**
What kind? _____	**Ventricular**
Conclusion: _____	**Accelerated idioventricular rhythm**

This accelerated idioventricular rhythm begins with an end-diastolic PVC, which is a fusion beat (fourth complex). There is an underlying sinus arrhythmia, and when the sinus rate slows to 55 beats/min, the accelerated ventricular focus manifests itself at a rate of 56 beats/min. A junctional escape mechanism is ruled out because of the fusion beat and the broad ventricular complexes.

Tracing 10-6

II

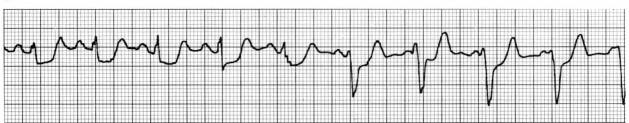

Rate: _____ beats/min   **80-88**

PR interval: _____ sec   **0.18**

QRS duration: _____ sec   **0.08**

QT interval: _____ sec   **0.38**

Ectopic beats? _____   **Yes**

What kind? _____   **Ventricular**

Conclusion: _____   **Accelerated**
                                             idioventricular
_____   **rhythm**

Here again, an accelerated idioventricular focus takes over as an end-diastolic PVC, which is a fusion beat (fourth complex). There are probably four more fusion beats before there is full capture of the ventricles by the ectopic focus.

Tracing 10-7

V₁

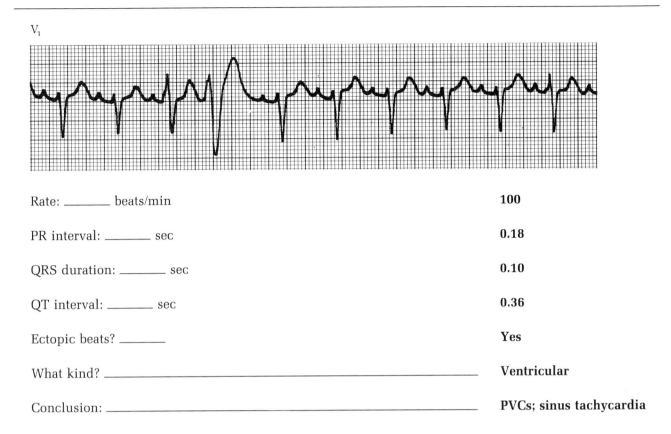

Rate: _____ beats/min   **100**

PR interval: _____ sec   **0.18**

QRS duration: _____ sec   **0.10**

QT interval: _____ sec   **0.36**

Ectopic beats? _____   **Yes**

What kind? _____   **Ventricular**

Conclusion: _____   **PVCs; sinus tachycardia**

There are two PVCs in this tracing. They are back to back, and the first of the pair is an end-diastolic fusion beat (third complex). A borderline sinus tachycardia is also present.

Tracing 10-8

II

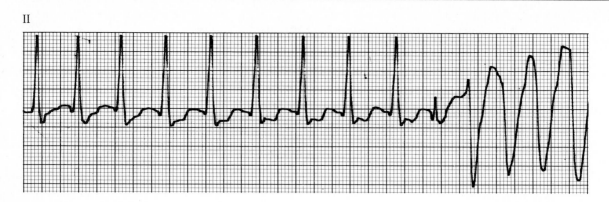

Rate: _____ beats/min

PR interval: _____ sec

QRS duration: _____ sec

QT interval: _____ sec

Ectopic beats? _____

What kind? _____

Conclusion: _____

_____

118-128 (underlying)

Indeterminable

0.16

Indeterminable

Yes

Ventricular

Supraventricular tachycardia and ventricular tachycardia

With only one tracing it is difficult to determine the mechanism of the underlying supraventricular tachycardia. A fusion beat toward the end of the tracing announces the onset of ventricular tachycardia (rate, 165 beats/min) and proves the supraventricular nature of the tachycardia preceding it.

Tracing 10-9

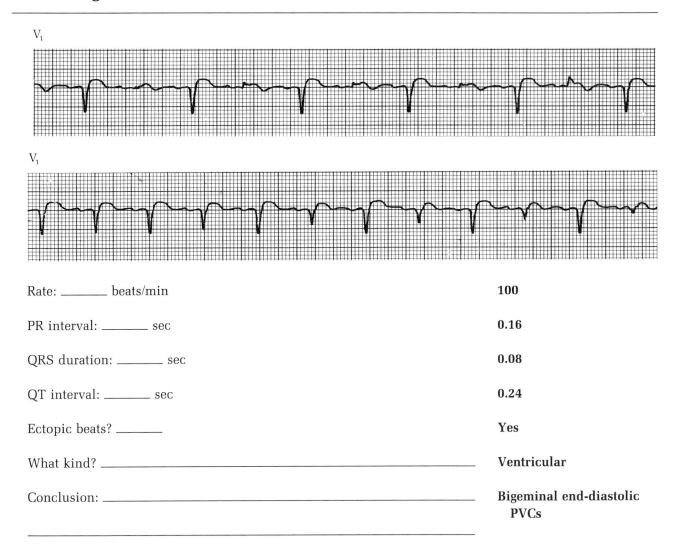

V₁

V₁

Rate: _____ beats/min	**100**
PR interval: _____ sec	**0.16**
QRS duration: _____ sec	**0.08**
QT interval: _____ sec	**0.24**
Ectopic beats? _____	**Yes**
What kind? _____	**Ventricular**
Conclusion: _____	**Bigeminal end-diastolic PVCs**

All of the bigeminal end-diastolic PVCs in this tracing are fusion beats, and they do not look like PVCs at all. Somebody might even mistake this tracing for electrical alternans. You can see the varying degrees of ventricular fusion every other beat, especially in the second tracing (from the same patient). The second beat in the tracing is a fusion, but it is not as apparent as the fourth beat. After this, every other complex has varying degrees of fusion until the complex is almost isoelectric. The only thing that can cause ventricular fusion in a sinus-conducted beat is a ventricular ectopic focus.

11
PARASYSTOLE

☐ **Classical parasystole and nonclassical parasystole**

☐ **Mechanism of entrance block**

Mechanism of ventricular parasystole

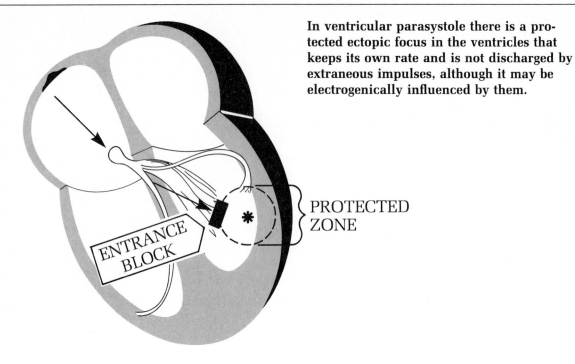

In ventricular parasystole there is a protected ectopic focus in the ventricles that keeps its own rate and is not discharged by extraneous impulses, although it may be electrogenically influenced by them.

PROTECTED ZONE

ENTRANCE BLOCK

In classical ventricular parasystole the rhythm of the ectopic focus is absolutely _____.

regular

Therefore the interectopic intervals will have a common _____.

denominator

The parasystolic focus does not always appear when expected, because the ventricles may be _____ as a result of activation by the sinus impulse.

refractory

Often the rhythm of the parasystolic focus is observed to be slightly irregular. This is because the extraneous _____ flowing around the protected area influence the rate of the ectopic focus.

currents

Classical ventricular parasystole

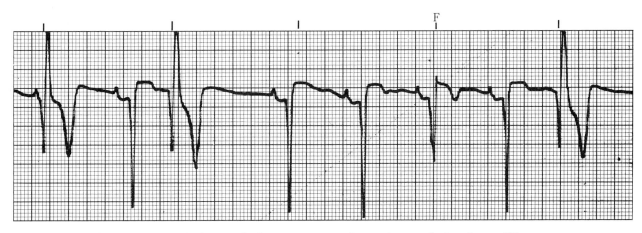

No fixed coupling interectopic intervals have common denominator fusion beats (*F*).

In ventricular parasystole the ectopic focus has its own undisturbed independent _____. **rhythm**

Therefore the ectopic beats will not be precisely _____ with a normal beat. **coupled**

Given a long enough tracing, there will eventually be a _____ beat. **fusion**

NOTE: *This is an unusual tracing in that all of the signs of parasystole are seen in a short segment. Usually a very long tracing is needed to demonstrate parasystole.*

Tracing 11-1

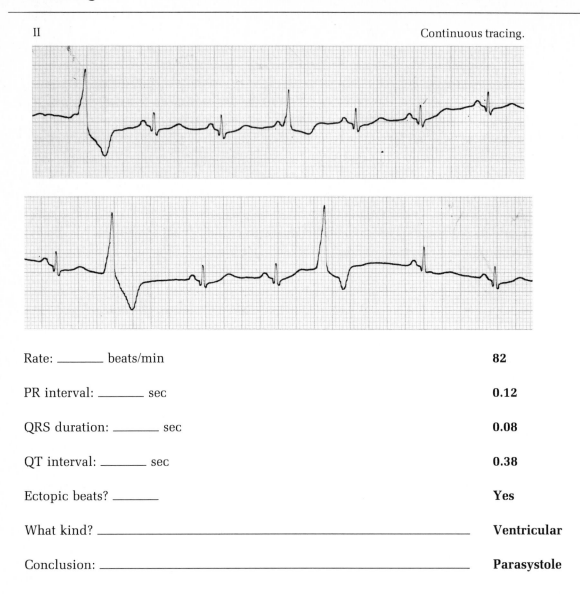

Rate: _____ beats/min   **82**

PR interval: _____ sec   **0.12**

QRS duration: _____ sec   **0.08**

QT interval: _____ sec   **0.38**

Ectopic beats? _____   **Yes**

What kind? _____   **Ventricular**

Conclusion: _____   **Parasystole**

The ventricular ectopics in this tracing are not exactly coupled to the preceding normal beats, and there is one fusion beat (the fourth). However, the interectopic intervals are not precise; for that reason, this is not a classical parasystole. Most parasystoles are not classical.

12

MYOCARDIAL INFARCTION

☐ **Subendocardial MI versus transmural MI**

☐ **Reflecting leads**

☐ **Reciprocal changes**

ECG changes in myocardial infarction

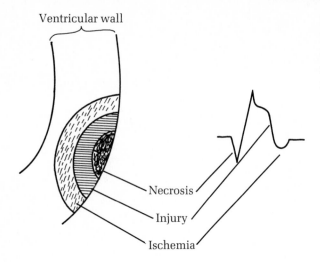

Ventricular wall

Necrosis

Injury

Ischemia

The diagnosis of myocardial infarction (MI) is made because of abnormal Q waves. The acute stage is reflected in elevated ST segments. Ischemia is reflected in symmetrical inverted T waves.

The infarcted tissue is electrically and physiologically dead. Therefore no currents flow toward the electrode over the infarct. This produces a pathological _____ wave on the ECG.

Q

A pathological Q wave is broader than _____ sec and 25% deeper than the R wave.

0.03

A fresh myocardial infarction is recognized because of _____ ST segments.

elevated

The T wave of ischemia is typically _____.

symmetrical

Subendocardial MI compared to transmural MI

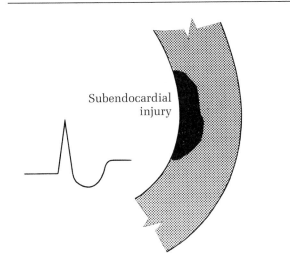

Subendocardial injury

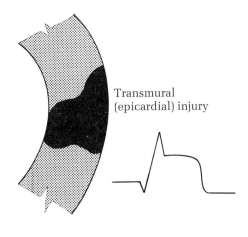

Transmural (epicardial) injury

In subendocardial myocardial infarction there are no _____ waves.   **Q**

In transmural myocardial infarction there are _____ waves.   **Q**

In subendocardial myocardial infarction the ST segment is _____.   **depressed**

In transmural myocardial infarction the ST segment is _____.   **elevated**

Reflecting leads

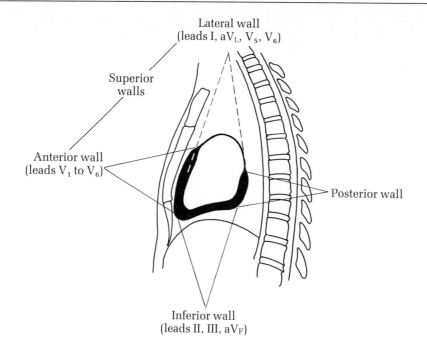

Lateral wall
(leads I, aV$_L$, V$_5$, V$_6$)

Superior
walls

Anterior wall
(leads V$_1$ to V$_6$)

Posterior wall

Inferior wall
(leads II, III, aV$_F$)

The heart has two main walls. They are _____ and _____.

inferior
superior

The leads reflecting the inferior wall are _____, _____, and _____.

II; III; aV$_F$

The leads reflecting the superior wall are all the remaining leads. They are _____, _____, and _____ to _____.

I; aV$_L$; V$_1$; V$_6$

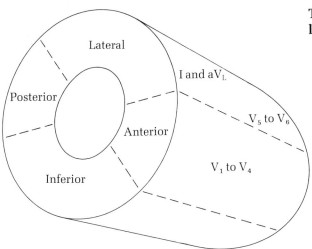

The superior wall has anterior and lateral aspects.

The left ventricle is shaped like a _____.

cylinder

Therefore the superior wall has _____ and _____ surfaces.

anterior; lateral

Leads _____ to _____ reflect the anterior wall.

V_1; V_4

Leads _____ and _____ reflect the lateral wall toward the apex.

V_5; V_6

Leads _____ and _____ reflect the lateral wall toward the base.

I; aV_L

Reciprocal changes

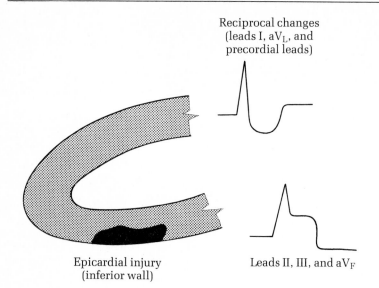

Reciprocal changes
(leads I, aV$_L$, and
precordial leads)

Epicardial injury
(inferior wall)

Leads II, III, and aV$_F$

The leads reflecting the wall opposite to the myocardial infarction will have changes opposite to those of the directly reflecting leads.

If there are elevated ST segments in the leads reflecting the inferior wall, there will be _____ ST segments in the leads reflecting the _____ wall.

depressed
superior

If there are elevated ST segments in the leads reflecting the anterior aspect of the superior wall, there will be _____ ST segments in the leads reflecting the inferior and/or lateral walls.

depressed

NOTE: Since the posterior wall has no electrodes over its surface, a myocardial infarction of that surface is reflected as reciprocal changes only in the anterior-wall leads.

Tracing 12-1

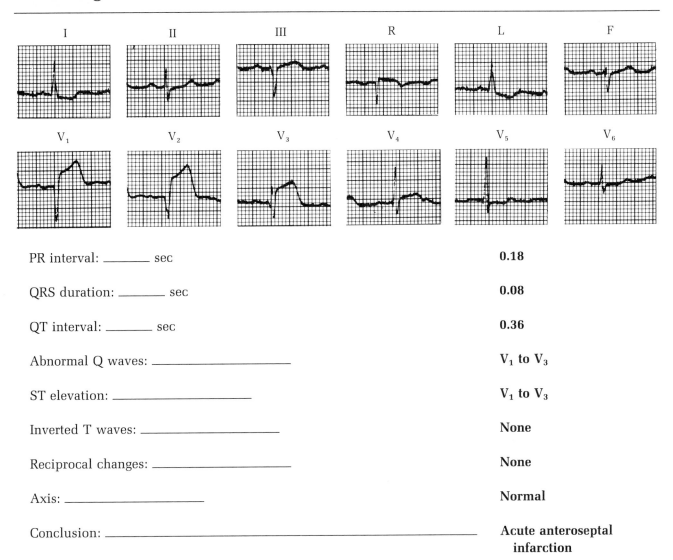

	I	II	III	R	L	F

| | V₁ | V₂ | V₃ | V₄ | V₅ | V₆ |

PR interval: _____ sec   **0.18**

QRS duration: _____ sec   **0.08**

QT interval: _____ sec   **0.36**

Abnormal Q waves: _____   **V₁ to V₃**

ST elevation: _____   **V₁ to V₃**

Inverted T waves: _____   **None**

Reciprocal changes: _____   **None**

Axis: _____   **Normal**

Conclusion: _____   **Acute anteroseptal
                                                                            infarction**

Tracing 12-2

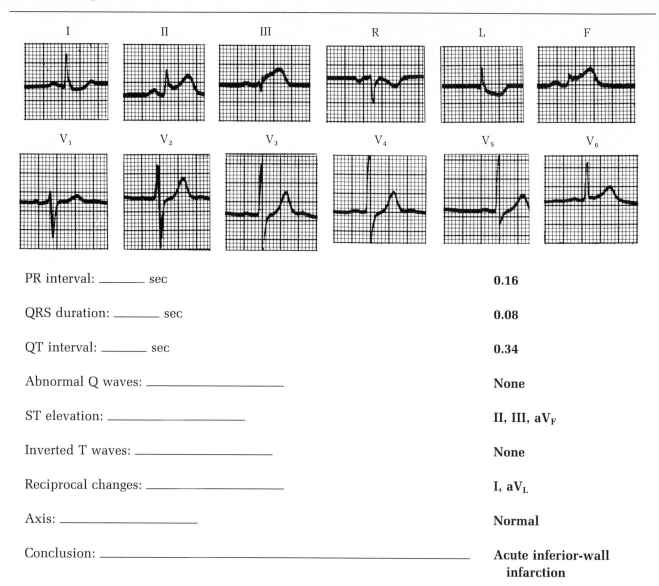

PR interval: _____ sec   **0.16**

QRS duration: _____ sec   **0.08**

QT interval: _____ sec   **0.34**

Abnormal Q waves: _____   **None**

ST elevation: _____   **II, III, aV$_F$**

Inverted T waves: _____   **None**

Reciprocal changes: _____   **I, aV$_L$**

Axis: _____   **Normal**

Conclusion: _____   **Acute inferior-wall infarction**

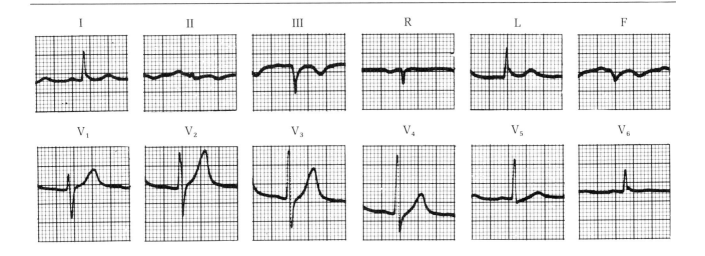

Eighteen days later (see ECG above) you can see the evolving pattern of an inferior infarction. In the inferior leads, where ST elevation was previously present, the ST segment has coved typically and the T waves have inverted. There are now QS waves in leads II and aV$_F$. At this stage in the evolution of the infarction, the nonfunctional tissue, reflected by the previous ST elevation, has either become necrotic (Q waves) or ischemic (T wave inversion).

Tracing 12-3

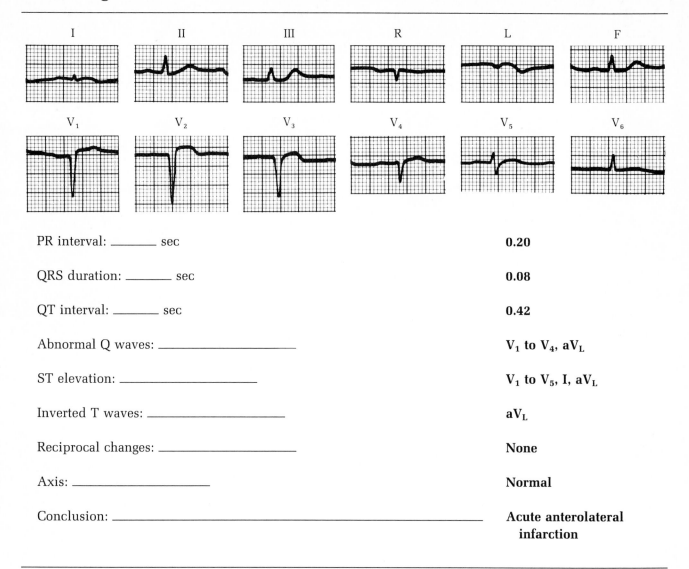

PR interval: _____ sec   **0.20**

QRS duration: _____ sec   **0.08**

QT interval: _____ sec   **0.42**

Abnormal Q waves: _____   **V_1 to V_4, aV_L**

ST elevation: _____   **V_1 to V_5, I, aV_L**

Inverted T waves: _____   **aV_L**

Reciprocal changes: _____   **None**

Axis: _____   **Normal**

Conclusion: _____   **Acute anterolateral infarction**

In this evolving anterolateral myocardial infarction the ST segments are still slightly elevated in the anterior chest leads (reflecting the anteroseptal area). There is evidence of extension to the lateral wall in the leads reflecting that surface. That is, there is coving of the ST segment in leads V_5, V_6, I, and aV_L, with T wave inversion in leads I and aV_L. Note that the loss of normal septal forces is not only reflected by the absence of r waves from leads V_1 to V_4 but also in the absence of normal little q waves in leads I and V_6.

As the healing process continues, the T waves in the anterior precordial leads will invert and become symmetrical and arrow shaped. This may also be the case in the leads reflecting the lateral wall.

Tracing 12-4

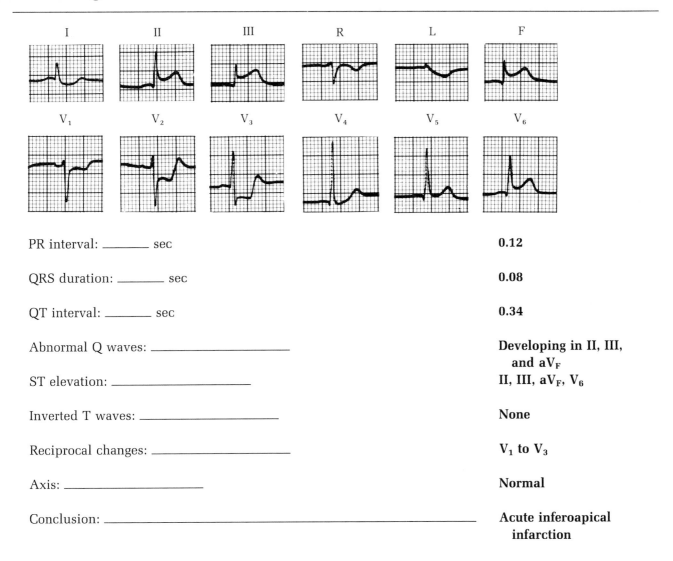

PR interval: _____ sec   **0.12**

QRS duration: _____ sec   **0.08**

QT interval: _____ sec   **0.34**

Abnormal Q waves: _____   **Developing in II, III, and aV$_F$**

ST elevation: _____   **II, III, aV$_F$, V$_6$**

Inverted T waves: _____   **None**

Reciprocal changes: _____   **V$_1$ to V$_3$**

Axis: _____   **Normal**

Conclusion: _____   **Acute inferoapical infarction**

There is ST segment elevation in the leads reflecting the inferior wall and the apex of the heart. Reciprocal changes can be seen in leads V$_1$ to V$_3$.

Tracing 12-5

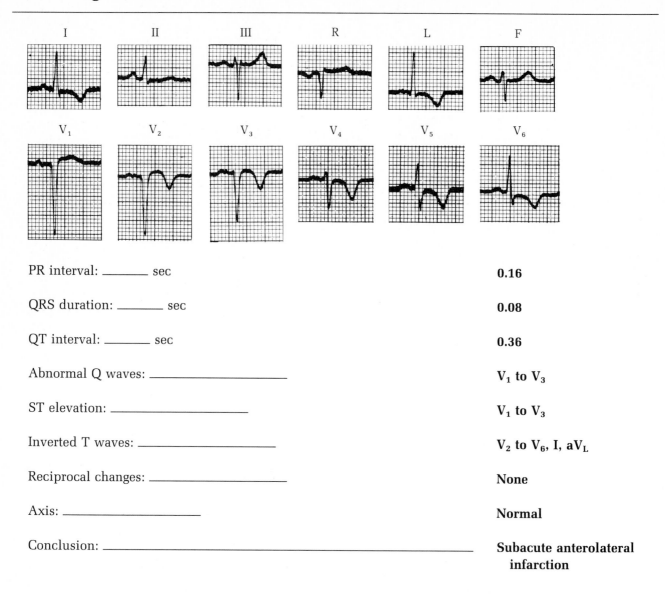

	I	II	III	R	L	F

	V₁	V₂	V₃	V₄	V₅	V₆

PR interval: _____ sec   **0.16**

QRS duration: _____ sec   **0.08**

QT interval: _____ sec   **0.36**

Abnormal Q waves: _____   **V₁ to V₃**

ST elevation: _____   **V₁ to V₃**

Inverted T waves: _____   **V₂ to V₆, I, aV_L**

Reciprocal changes: _____   **None**

Axis: _____   **Normal**

Conclusion: _____   **Subacute anterolateral infarction**

This is a subacute (evolving) anteroseptal myocardial infarction, with involvement of the lateral wall. The acute sign of infarction (ST elevation) has evolved into T wave inversion with a typical arrow shape to the T waves. The ST segments in the leads reflecting the anterior and lateral walls are typically coved upward.

Tracing 12-6

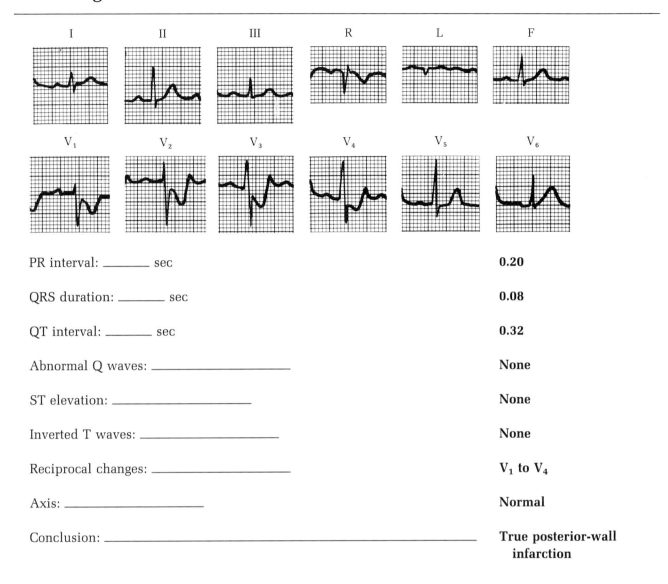

PR interval: _____ sec   **0.20**

QRS duration: _____ sec   **0.08**

QT interval: _____ sec   **0.32**

Abnormal Q waves: _____   **None**

ST elevation: _____   **None**

Inverted T waves: _____   **None**

Reciprocal changes: _____   **V₁ to V₄**

Axis: _____   **Normal**

Conclusion: _____   **True posterior-wall infarction**

In this ECG showing of an acute posterior-wall infarction, you have the opportunity to see changes that are purely reciprocal. This is because none of the routine 12 leads faces this surface of the heart. However, the leads on the opposite side of the heart will reflect reciprocal changes (anterior leads). That is, instead of abnormal Q waves and ST elevation, there will be an increase in the height and width of the R waves and ST depression, especially in leads V_1 and V_2.

Tracing 12-7

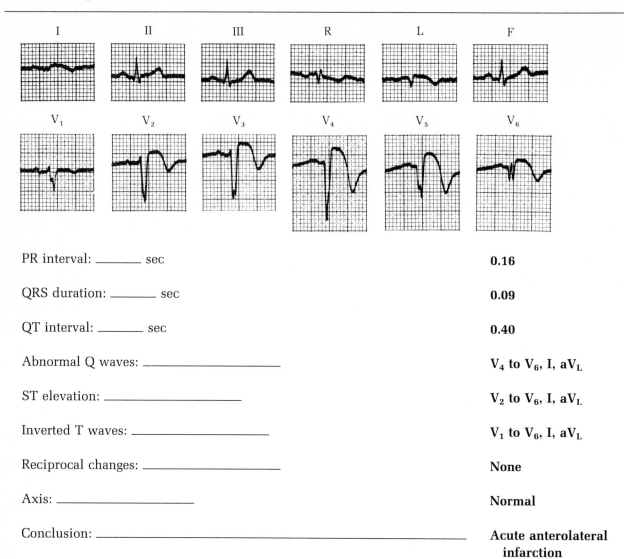

PR interval: _____ sec   **0.16**

QRS duration: _____ sec   **0.09**

QT interval: _____ sec   **0.40**

Abnormal Q waves: _____   **V_4 to V_6, I, aV_L**

ST elevation: _____   **V_2 to V_6, I, aV_L**

Inverted T waves: _____   **V_1 to V_6, I, aV_L**

Reciprocal changes: _____   **None**

Axis: _____   **Normal**

Conclusion: _____   **Acute anterolateral infarction**

13

CHAMBER ENLARGEMENT

- ☐ **Left-ventricular hypertrophy**
- ☐ **Left-atrial enlargement**
- ☐ **P-mitrale**
- ☐ **Right-ventricular hypertrophy**
- ☐ **Right-atrial enlargement**
- ☐ **P-pulmonale**

Left-ventricular hypertrophy

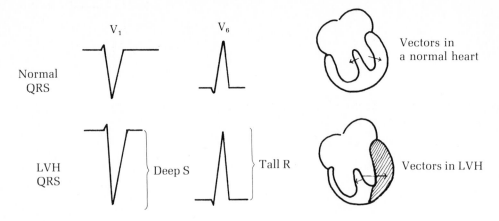

In left-ventricular hypertrophy there is a further disproportion in size between the left and right ventricles.

Thus leads over the left ventricle have taller _____ waves.   **R**

Leads over the right ventricle have deeper _____ waves.   **S**

NOTE: *Criteria for the ECG diagnosis of left-ventricular hypertrophy are plagued with false positives. It is important to evaluate the total clinical picture of the patient before making judgments regarding the ECG finding of left-ventricular hypertrophy.*

Left-atrial enlargement

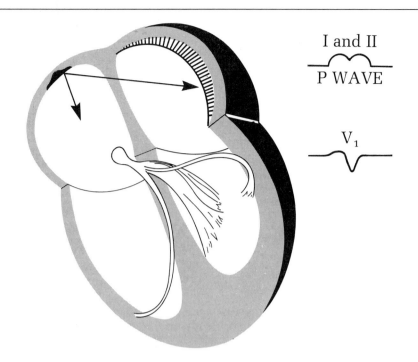

I and II

P WAVE

V_1

P-mitrale.

Left-atrial enlargement produces an M-shaped P in leads _____ and _____ and a deep broad terminal trough in lead _____.

I

II; V_1

Left-atrial enlargement may be associated with left-ventricular _____.

hypertrophy

Right-ventricular hypertrophy

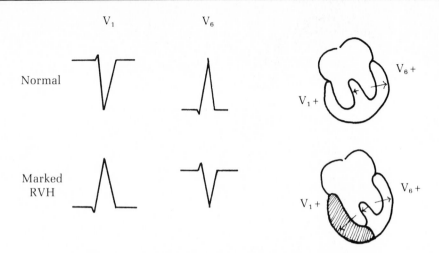

Before the typical pattern is manifested, there is a significant
degree of hypertrophy. Normally the left ventricle is about three times
thicker than the right; thus, as the right ventricle becomes thicker,
it begins to balance out anterior and posterior electrical forces
before it actually dominates.

As the right ventricle hypertrophies, the QRS voltage in V_1 is _____ **reduced**
before an R wave actually appears.

Right axis deviation is an important ECG sign of right-ventricular
_____. **hypertrophy**

In fully developed right-ventricular hypertrophy the R in V_1 is greater than
the _____, and the R in V_6 is smaller than the _____. **S; S**

Right-atrial enlargement

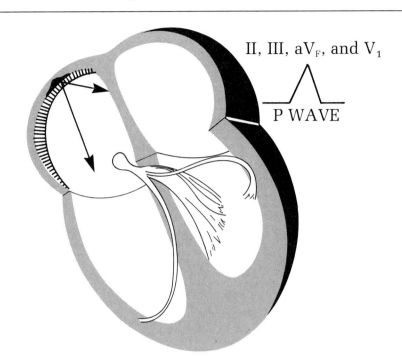

II, III, aV$_F$, and V$_1$

P WAVE

In right-atrial enlargement there are tall peaked P waves in leads _____, _____, _____, and sometimes _____.

II
III; aV$_F$; V$_1$

Tracing 13-1

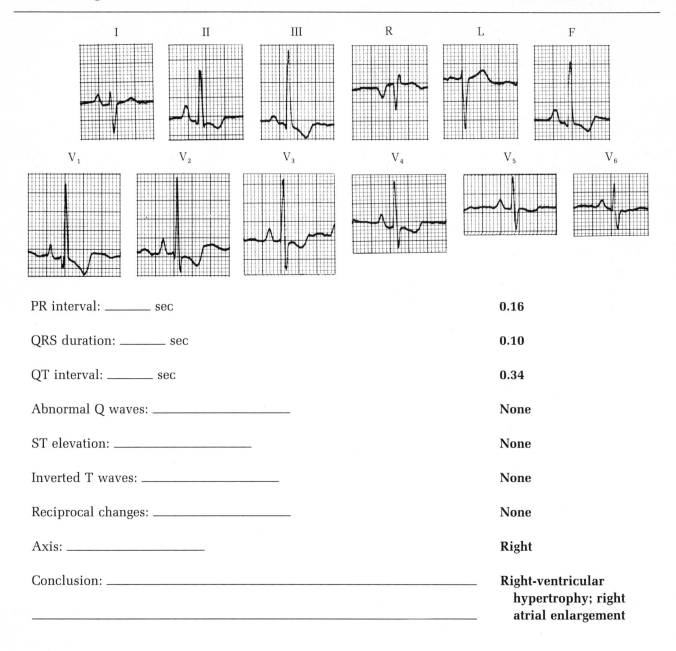

| I | II | III | R | L | F |

| V₁ | V₂ | V₃ | V₄ | V₅ | V₆ |

PR interval: _____ sec   **0.16**

QRS duration: _____ sec   **0.10**

QT interval: _____ sec   **0.34**

Abnormal Q waves: _____   **None**

ST elevation: _____   **None**

Inverted T waves: _____   **None**

Reciprocal changes: _____   **None**

Axis: _____   **Right**

Conclusion: _____   **Right-ventricular**
_____   **hypertrophy; right**
                                                            atrial enlargement

---

    Because of the prominent R wave in lead V_1, this ECG must be differentiated from true posterior myocardial infarction. When right axis deviation and right-atrial enlargement (note the tall, pointed P waves) accompany such a morphology in lead V_1, the diagnosis of right-ventricular hypertrophy (RVH) is more likely. Minimal QRS prolongation is seen, probably reflective of incomplete RBBB, which is sometimes additional evidence of RVH.

Tracing 13-2

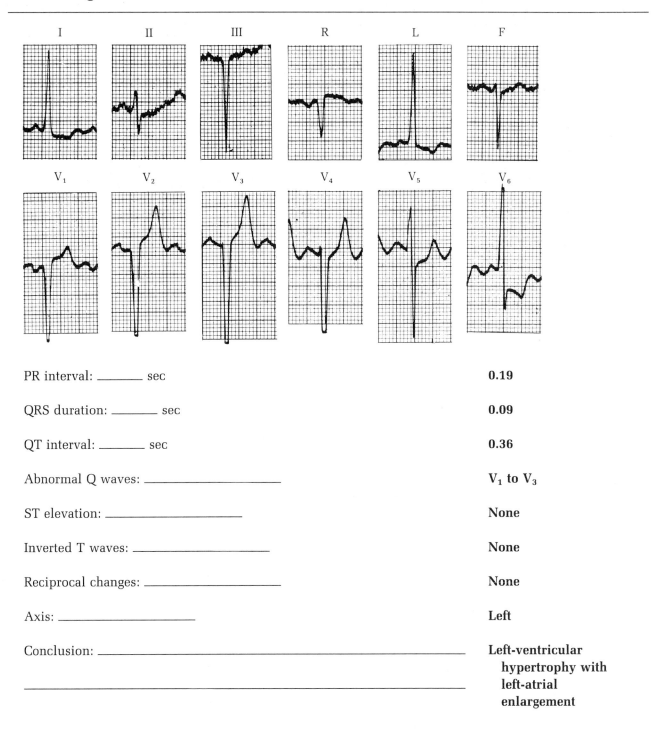

PR interval: _____ sec   **0.19**

QRS duration: _____ sec   **0.09**

QT interval: _____ sec   **0.36**

Abnormal Q waves: _____   **V_1 to V_3**

ST elevation: _____   **None**

Inverted T waves: _____   **None**

Reciprocal changes: _____   **None**

Axis: _____   **Left**

Conclusion: _____   **Left-ventricular**
_____   **hypertrophy with**
                                                   left-atrial
                                                 enlargement

This ECG represents left-ventricular hypertrophy (LVH). It may be confused with myocardial infarction because of poor R wave progression (QS complexes from V_1 to V_3). Anteroseptal myocardial infarction may also be present, however. A vectorcardiogram may be helpful in distinguishing between the two.

Tracing 13-3

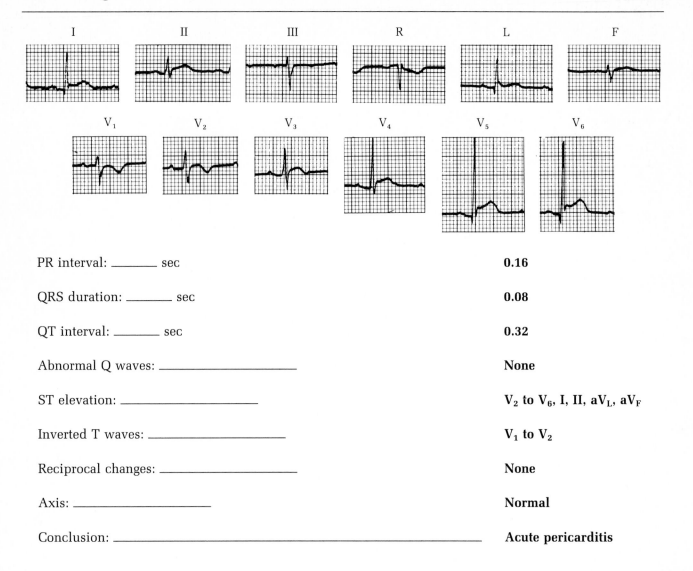

PR interval: _____ sec   **0.16**

QRS duration: _____ sec   **0.08**

QT interval: _____ sec   **0.32**

Abnormal Q waves: _____   **None**

ST elevation: _____   **V$_2$ to V$_6$, I, II, aV$_L$, aV$_F$**

Inverted T waves: _____   **V$_1$ to V$_2$**

Reciprocal changes: _____   **None**

Axis: _____   **Normal**

Conclusion: _____   **Acute pericarditis**

Acute pericarditis must be differentiated from acute myocardial infarction because of the elevated ST segments seen in the limb leads and left precordial leads and because of T wave inversion.

In acute pericarditis the ST segment elevation is not accompanied by reciprocal ST depression. For example, in the above tracing there is ST elevation in both leads I and III. The shape of the ST segment in pericarditis is typically concave instead of convex, as in myocardial infarction. The ECG of pericarditis evolves quickly, within a few weeks, and Q *waves will not appear.*

Characteristically the ST segments in acute pericarditis will be elevated in many leads with upright T waves except in lead III, where the T waves may be inverted. After this the ST segment becomes isoelectric, and there is widespread T wave inversion. The ST and T wave changes take place in the course of several weeks.

14

PACEMAKERS

- ☐ **VVI**
- ☐ **AAI**
- ☐ **VDD**
- ☐ **DVI**
- ☐ **DDD**

This chapter was written in collaboration with Anita Powe, Clinical
Administrative Manager, Telectronics, Englewood, Colorado.

Confused with new pacemaker terminology?

The uncomplicated days of simple terms such as "QRS inhibited" and "QRS triggered" pacemakers are gone forever. The new multifaceted programmability of pacemakers has brought with it a multiplicity of abbreviations. For example, the new DDD system has the potential of pacing both the atrium and the ventricle, sensing both, being inhibited by an intrinsic or paced complex from either chamber, and triggering a ventricular response to intrinsic atrial activity. In addition, at any time this system is capable of operating in any of four other modes (VVI, AAI, VDD, and DVI), which are discussed in the following pages.

The first step in understanding the new pacemakers is to familarize yourself with the concept implied by each abbreviation. No one in critical care today needs to define "PVC" or "PAC." You know in a conceptual way what those terms imply not only arrhythmogenically but also clinically. You must achieve the same facility with the pacemaker code; the best way to do so is simply to use the code until it becomes as natural to you as "QRS," "PR," or "PVC."

The three-letter code

ICHD CODE:

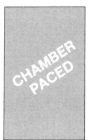 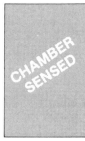 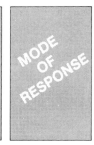

The first and second letters can be *V* (ventricle), *A* (atrium), or *D* (dual, both atrium and ventricle). The third letter can be *I* (inhibited), *T* (triggered), or *D* (dual response, either inhibited or triggered).

The first letter describes the ＿＿＿＿＿＿ chamber.   **paced**

The second letter describes the ＿＿＿＿＿＿ chamber.   **sensed**

The third letter describes the ＿＿＿＿＿ ＿＿＿ ＿＿＿＿＿＿.   **mode of response**
   I = ＿＿＿＿＿＿＿＿＿   **inhibited**
   T = ＿＿＿＿＿＿＿＿＿   **triggered**

If only the ventricle is being paced and sensed and the pacer is inhibited by a QRS, the system is ＿＿＿.   **VVI**

If only the atrium is being paced and sensed and the pacer is inhibited by a P wave, the system is ＿＿＿.   **AAI**

If only the ventricle is being paced but both chambers are being sensed and the pacer is triggered by an intrinsic P wave or inhibited by an intrinsic QRS, the system is ＿＿＿.   **VDD**

If both chambers are being paced but sensing occurs only in the ventricle and the pacer is inhibited by a QRS, the system is ＿＿＿.   **DVI**

If both chambers are being paced and sensed and the pacer is inhibited by a P or QRS and triggered by a QRS, the system is ＿＿＿.   **DDD**

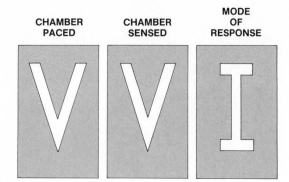

| CHAMBER PACED | CHAMBER SENSED | MODE OF RESPONSE |

V, Ventricle; *I,* inhibited. In VVI pacing there is only one chamber to evaluate— the ventricle.

A VVI pacemaker paces and senses only in the _____.   **ventricle**

The mode of response is _____.   **inhibited**

The VVI unit is inhibited by intrinsic _____ activity.   **ventricular**

This type of pacing is not physiological because there is no relationship between intrinsic _____ activity and paced _____ activity.   **atrial; ventricular**

CHAMBER PACED	CHAMBER SENSED	MODE OF RESPONSE
A	A	I

A, Atrium; *I*, inhibited.

An AAI pacemaker both paces and senses only in the _____. **atrium**

The mode of response is _____. **inhibited**

The AAI unit is inhibited by intrinsic _____ activity. **atrial**

This type of pacing is physiological because it paces the _____ **atrium**
and assumes intact _____ conduction. **AV**

CHAMBER PACED	CHAMBER SENSED	MODE OF RESPONSE

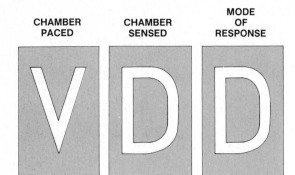

V, Ventricle; *D,* dual (dual-chamber sensing and dual mode of response—inhibited and triggered).

The VDD pacemaker paces the _____ but senses in _____ _____. **ventricle** **both chambers**

The VDD unit is triggered by intrinsic _____ activity or inhibited by intrinsic _____ activity. **atrial** **ventricular**

The VDD unit is not always physiological because it will pace only the _____ when there is no intrinsic atrial or ventricular activity. **ventricle**

290

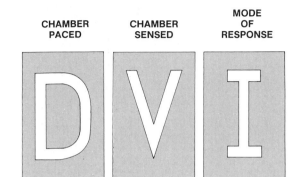

CHAMBER PACED	CHAMBER SENSED	MODE OF RESPONSE
D	V	I

D, Dual; *V*, ventricle; *I*, inhibited. In the committed DVI system, paced atrial activity is always followed by a ventricular output spike. In the noncommitted DVI system, ventricular activity following a paced or intrinsic atrial event is sensed and the pacemaker inhibited.

The DVI pacemaker may pace in _____ _____, but sensing occurs only in the _____.

both chambers
ventricle

DVI pacing is physiological because _____ pacing occurs when there is no intrinsic ventricular activity.

atrial

In the committed DVI system the ventricle will alway be paced following an _____ paced beat even though it is followed by an intrinsic ventricular beat.

atrial

The DVI system will pace the atrium and ventricle even though there is intrinsic atrial activity, because the unit does not _____ atrial activity.

sense

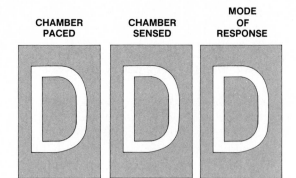

CHAMBER PACED   CHAMBER SENSED   MODE OF RESPONSE

D, Dual (dual-chamber pacing and sensing and dual mode of response. In DDD pacing both chambers must be evaluated.

The DDD system paces and senses in either chamber or _____ _____.   **both chambers**

The DDD system inhibits in either chamber or _____ _____, and intrinsic atrial activity will result in a triggered _____ response.   **both chambers ventricular**

The DDD system operates in the DVI mode when it _____ both chambers and when intrinsic atrial and ventricular activity _____ the pacer.   **paces inhibits**

The DDD system operates in the AAI mode when a paced _____ complex is followed by an _____ ventricular one.   **atrial intrinsic**

The DDD system operates in the _____ mode when sensed atrial activity is followed by paced ventricular activity.   **VDD**

Tracing 14-1

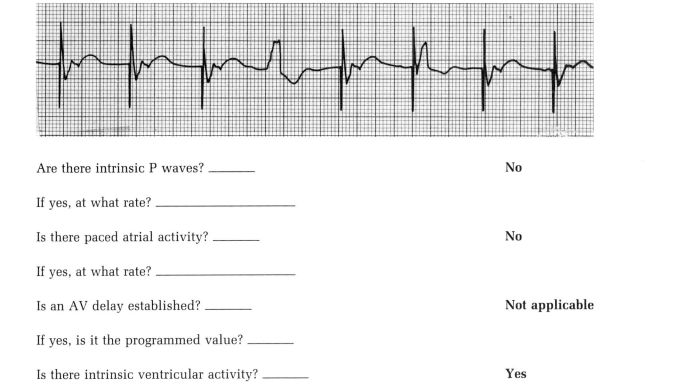

Are there intrinsic P waves? _____   **No**

If yes, at what rate? _____

Is there paced atrial activity? _____   **No**

If yes, at what rate? _____

Is an AV delay established? _____   **Not applicable**

If yes, is it the programmed value? _____

Is there intrinsic ventricular activity? _____   **Yes**

If yes, was it sensed? _____   **Yes**

Is there paced ventricular activity? _____   **Yes**

If yes, at what rate? _____   **75 ppm**

Conclusion: _____   **Normally functioning VVI pacemaker**

This is a VVI pacemaker; that is, both sensing and pacing occur in the ventricle, and the pacemaker is inhibited by intrinsic ventricular activity. Ventricular pacing occurs at a rate of 75 pulses per minute (ppm). Note the ventricular ectopic beat (fourth complex is sensed and the pacemaker inhibited). This patient evidently has an underlying ventricular parasystole (ventricular ectopic activity with no fixed coupling). There are two ventricular ectopic beats in this tracing; one is sensed and the pacemaker is inhibited; the other (sixth complex) is not sensed because it falls during the refractory period of the pacemaker. It is a fusion beat; that is, the ventricular ectopic focus discharged just after the pacemaker impulse, causing the two currents to collide.

Of interest are the retrograde P waves following the ventricular paced beats. Because this pacemaker does not sense atrial activity, they are of no concern.

293

Tracing 14-2

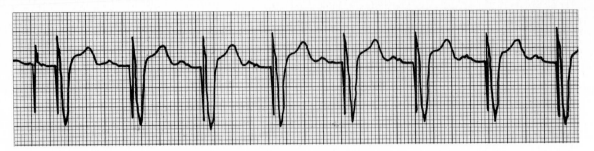

Programmed parameters: DDD; ventricular rate, 60 ppm; AV delay, 230 msec.

Are there intrinsic P waves? _____	**Yes**
If yes, at what rate? _____	**75 beats/min**
Is there paced atrial activity? _____	**Yes**
If yes, at what rate? _____	**Indeterminable**
Is an AV delay established? _____	**Yes**
If yes, is it the programmed value? _____	**Yes**
Is there intrinsic ventricular activity? _____	**No**
If yes, was it sensed? _____	
Is there paced ventricular activity? _____	**Yes**
If yes, at what rate? _____	**77 ppm**
Conclusion: _____	**Normally functioning DDD pacemaker**

Sensing and pacing are occurring in both the atrium and the ventricle. In the first complex the atrium is paced; there follows the programmed AV delay of 230 msec, following which the ventricle is paced. In the rest of the tracing the unit is functioning normally in the VDD mode because there is intrinsic atrial activity (note the P waves). This intrinsic atrial activity is sensed, and at the onset of the P wave an AV delay is initiated. Since in this patient no intrinsic ventricular activity is sensed, the ventricles are paced at the end of the AV delay. There is ventricular tracking of intrinsic atrial activity.

Tracing 14-3

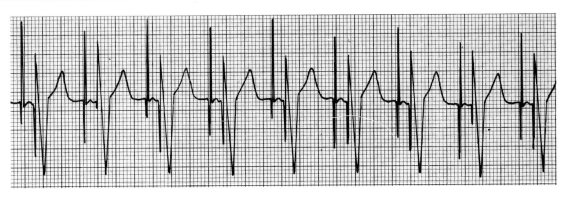

Programmed parameters: DDD; ventricular rate, 88 ppm; AV delay, 140 msec.

Are there intrinsic P waves? _____   **No**

If yes, at what rate? _____

Is there paced atrial activity? _____   **Yes**

If yes, at what rate? _____   **88 ppm**

Is an AV delay established? _____   **Yes**

If yes, is it the programmed value? _____   **Yes**

Is there intrinsic ventricular activity? _____   **No**

If yes, was it sensed? _____

Is there paced ventricular activity? _____   **Yes**

If yes, at what rate? _____   **88 ppm**

Conclusion: _____   **DDD pacemaker**
_____   **functioning in the**
          DVI mode

Pacing is occurring in both the atrium and the ventricle. There is no evidence of intrinsic activity.

Tracing 14-4

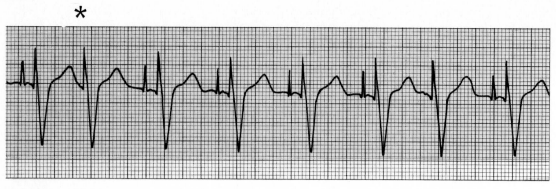

Programmed parameters: DDD; ventricular rate, 75 ppm; AV delay, 140 msec.

Are there intrinsic P waves? _____ **Yes**

If yes, at what rate? _____ **Indeterminable**

Is there paced atrial activity? _____ **Yes**

If yes, at what rate? _____ **75 ppm**

Is an AV delay established? _____ **Yes**

If yes, is it the programmed value? _____ **Yes**

Is there intrinsic ventricular activity? _____ **No**

If yes, was it sensed? _____

Is there paced ventricular activity? _____ **Yes**

If yes, at what rate? _____ **75 ppm**

Conclusion: _____ **Normally functioning DDD pacemaker**

_____

The complexes marked with asterisks indicate sensing of intrinsic atrial activity. An AV delay is initiated and the ventricle is paced, since no intrinsic ventricular activity occurs. In all other complexes, no atrial activity is sensed; therefore the atrium is paced.

Tracing 14-5

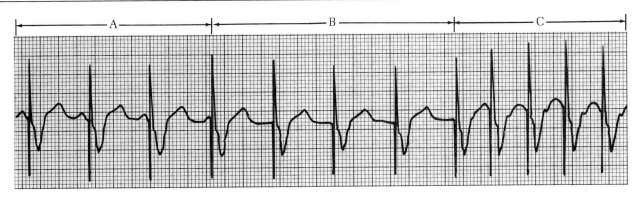

Programmed parameters: VDD; ventricular rate, 90 ppm; AV delay, 110 msec; maximal ventricular rate, 150 ppm.

Are there intrinsic P waves? _____	**Yes**
If yes, at what rate? _____	**90 to 150 beats/min**
Is there paced atrial activity? _____	**No**
If yes, at what rate? _____	
Is an AV delay established? _____	**Yes**
If yes, is it the programmed value? _____	**Yes**
Is there intrinsic ventricular activity? _____	**No**
If yes, was it sensed? _____	
Is there paced ventricular activity? _____	**Yes**
If yes, at what rate? _____	**90 to 150 ppm**
Conclusion: _____	**Normally functioning VDD pacemaker**

In section A, the pacemaker is tracking the P waves at a rate of approximately 90 ppm. In section B, there is no apparent atrial activity; therefore the ventricles are paced at the programmed rate of 90 ppm. In section C, atrial activity is sensed at a rate greater than the maximal ventricular rate of 150 ppm; therefore the pacemaker will only pace at a rate of 150 ppm.

Tracing 14-6

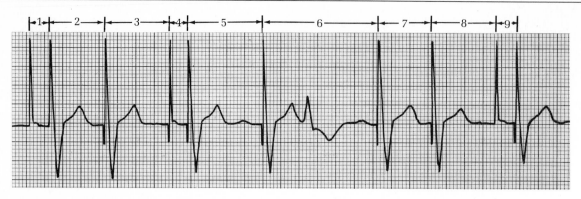

Programmed parameters: DDD; ventricular rate, 65 ppm; AV delay, 200 msec.

Are there intrinsic P waves? _____   **Yes**

If yes, at what rate? _____   **Indeterminable**

Is there paced atrial activity? _____   **Yes**

If yes, at what rate? _____   **Erratic**

Is an AV delay established? _____   **Yes**

If yes, is it the programmed value? _____   **Yes**

Is there intrinsic ventricular activity? _____   **Yes**

If yes, was it sensed? _____   **Yes**

Is there paced ventricular activity? _____   **Yes**

If yes, at what rate? _____   **65 ppm**

Conclusion: _____   **Normally functioning DDD pacemaker**

_____

The numbers below refer to those above the tracing.

1. AV delay is 200 msec, as programmed; the ventricle is paced
2. P wave (hidden in T) is sensed and the ventricle is paced
3. VA interval (720 msec), during which no intrinsic activity is sensed, causes atrium to be paced
4. AV delay, ventricle paced
5. P wave sensed during VA interval; no R wave sensed, so the ventricle is paced
6. PVC sensed, VA interval reset, P wave sensed, no R wave; therefore the ventricle is paced
7. P wave (in the T) is sensed; ventricle is paced
8. VA interval, no P wave sensed, atrium paced
9. AV delay, no R wave sensed, ventricle paced, DDD mode; there is pacing in both the atrium and the ventricle

Tracing 14-7

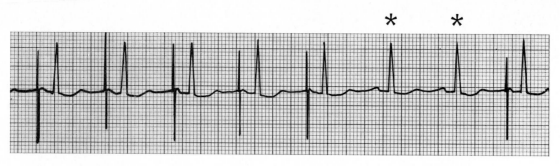

Programmed parameters: DDD; ventricular rate, 75 ppm; AV delay, 230 msec.

Are there intrinsic P waves? _____	**Yes**
If yes, at what rate? _____	**87 beats/min**
Is there paced atrial activity? _____	**Yes**
If yes, at what rate? _____	**80 ppm**
Is an AV delay established? _____	**Yes**
If yes, is it the programmed value? _____	**Yes**
Is there intrinsic ventricular activity? _____	**Yes**
If yes, was it sensed? _____	**Yes**
Is there paced ventricular activity? _____	**No**
If yes, at what rate? _____	
Conclusion: _____ _____	**DDD pacemaker functioning in the AAI mode**

There is an atrial spike prior to each of the first five intrinsic ventricular complexes. The next two R waves (*asterisks*) are preceded by intrinsic atrial activity (P waves), which arrive prior to the expiration of the VA interval and inhibit the pacemaker. The atrium is being paced only when no intrinsic atrial activity is sensed.

Tracing 14-8

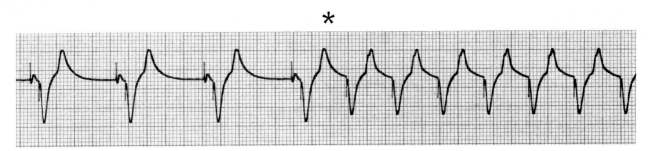

*

Programmed parameters: DDD; ventricular rate; 60 ppm; AV delay, 120 msec.

Are there intrinsic P waves? _____ **No**

If yes, at what rate? _____

Is there paced atrial activity? _____ **Yes**

If yes, at what rate? _____ **60 ppm**

Is an AV delay established? _____ **Yes**

If yes, is it the programmed value? _____ **Yes**

Is there intrinsic ventricular activity? _____ **No**

If yes, was it sensed? _____

Is there paced ventricular activity? _____ **Yes**

If yes, at what rate? _____ **60 ppm**

Conclusion: _____ **Pacemaker-mediated**
_____ **endless-loop**
tachycardia

This DDD pacemaker does not have a long enough programmed atrial refractory period, since a retrograde P wave from a paced ventricular beat (asterisk) activates the ventricular pacemaker and a pacemaker-mediated endless-loop tachycardia is initiated. Each time the ventricle is depolarized by the pacemaker stimulus, the impulse is retrogradely conducted into the right atrium and is subsequently detected by the the atrial electrode. The pulse generator then triggers the next ventricular stimulus, and the cycle is repeated over and over. One way to terminate such a tachycardia is to switch to a DVI mode, thus eliminating atrial sensing.

Tracing 14-9

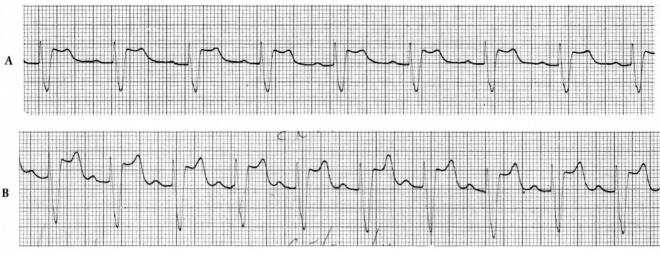

A

B

Programmed parameters: DDD; ventricular rate, 60 ppm; AV delay, 230 msec.
(Courtesy Dr. John H.K. Vogel, Santa Barbara, Calif.)

Are there intrinsic P waves? _____	**Yes**
If yes, at what rate? _____	**A, 74 beats/min; B, 88 beats/min**
Is there paced atrial activity? _____	**No**
If yes, at what rate? _____	
Is an AV delay established? _____	**Yes**
If yes, is it the programmed value? _____	**Yes**
Is there intrinsic ventricular activity? _____	**No**
If yes, was it sensed? _____	
Is there paced ventricular activity? _____	**Yes**
If yes, at what rate? _____	**A, 74 ppm; B, 88 ppm**
Conclusion: _____	**Normally functioning DDD pacemaker**

The intrinsic atrial activity (sinus P waves) is being sensed, and, after a programmed AV delay of 230 msec, the ventricle is paced. With exercise *(B)*, the sinus rate increases to 88 beats/min. This increased intrinsic atrial rate is sensed, and the ventricle is paced accordingly.

Appendix

Normal QT intervals and the upper limits of the normal

Heart rate (beats/min)	Men and children (sec)	Women (sec)	Upper limits of the normal	
			Men and children (sec)	Women (sec)
40.0	0.449	0.461	0.491	0.503
43.0	0.438	0.450	0.479	0.491
46.0	0.426	0.438	0.466	0.478
48.0	0.420	0.432	0.460	0.471
50.0	0.414	0.425	0.453	0.464
52.0	0.407	0.418	0.445	0.456
54.5	0.400	0.411	0.438	0.449
57.0	0.393	0.404	0.430	0.441
60.0	0.386	0.396	0.422	0.432
63.0	0.378	0.388	0.413	0.423
66.5	0.370	0.380	0.404	0.414
70.5	0.361	0.371	0.395	0.405
75.0	0.352	0.362	0.384	0.394
80.0	0.342	0.352	0.374	0.384
86.0	0.332	0.341	0.363	0.372
92.5	0.321	0.330	0.351	0.360
100.0	0.310	0.318	0.338	0.347
109.0	0.297	0.305	0.325	0.333
120.0	0.283	0.291	0.310	0.317
133.0	0.268	0.276	0.294	0.301
150.0	0.252	0.258	0.275	0.282
172.0	0.234	0.240	0.255	0.262

From Ashman, R., and Hull, E.: Essentials of electrocardiography, New York, 1945, Macmillan, Inc. Reproduced with the kind permission of Edgar Hull, M.D.